Patient
Communication for
Pharmacy

A Case-Study Approach on Theory and Practice

Min Liu, PhD, MPH
Associate Professor
Department of Applied Communication Studies
Southern Illinois University Edwardsville

Lakesha M. Butler, PharmD, BCPS
Clinical Associate Professor
Department of Pharmacy Practice, School of Pharmacy
Southern Illinois University Edwardsville

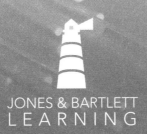

JONES & BARTLETT
LEARNING

World Headquarters
Jones & Bartlett Learning
5 Wall Street
Burlington, MA 01803
978-443-5000
info@jblearning.com
www.jblearning.com

Jones & Bartlett Learning books and products are available through most bookstores and online booksellers. To contact Jones & Bartlett Learning directly, call 800-832-0034, fax 978-443-8000, or visit our website, www. jblearning.com.

Substantial discounts on bulk quantities of Jones & Bartlett Learning publications are available to corporations, professional associations, and other qualified organizations. For details and specific discount information, contact the special sales department at Jones & Bartlett Learning via the above contact information or send an email to specialsales@jblearning.com.

8213-2

Production Credits

Chief Executive Officer: Ty Field
President: James Homer
Chief Product Officer: Eduardo Moura
Publisher: Cathy L. Esperti
Editorial Assistant: Sara J. Peterson
Production Editor: Sarah Vostok
Marketing Manager: Grace Richards
VP, Manufacturing and
  Inventory Control: Therese Connell
Composition: Integra Software Services Pvt. Ltd.
Cover Design: Scott Moden
Rights & Media Research Coordinator: Jamey O'Quinn
Media Development Editor: Shannon Sheehan
Cover Image: © Dostoevsky / Shutterstock
Printing and Binding: Edwards Brothers Malloy
Cover Printing: Edwards Brothers Malloy

Library of Congress Cataloging-in-Publication Data

Liu, Min, 1977- , author.
  Patient communication for pharmacy : a case-study approach on theory and practice / Min Liu and Lakesha M. Butler.
    p. ; cm.
  Includes bibliographical references.
  ISBN 978-1-284-03888-0
  I. Butler, Lakesha M., author. II. Title.
  [DNLM: 1. Health Communication. 2. Pharmacists–standards. 3. Clinical Competence. 4. Cultural Competency. 5. Professional-Patient Relations–ethics. QV 21]
  RS56
  615.1–dc23
                        2015028794

6048

Printed in the United States of America
20 19 18 17 16   10 9 8 7 6 5 4 3 2 1

TABLE OF CONTENTS

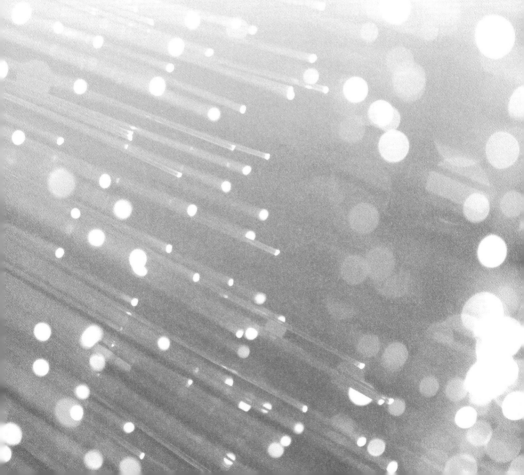

I dedicate this book to my loving parents, who taught me the value of reading and learning.

Min Liu

I dedicate this book to my wonderful family and friends for all of their love and support, and to all of my patients, who have made me a better pharmacist.

Lakesha M. Butler

CONTRIBUTORS

Chapter 4
Kelly N. Gable, PharmD, BCPP
Associate Professor
School of Pharmacy
Southern Illinois University Edwardsville

Chapter 9
Miranda Nelson, PharmD
Pediatric Antimicrobial Stewardship Pharmacist
St. Louis Children's Hospital

Chapter 10
J. Mark Ruscin, PharmD, FCCP, BCPS
Professor and Department Chair, Pharmacy Practice
School of Pharmacy
Southern Illinois University Edwardsville

FOREWORD

PHARMACIST–PATIENT COMMUNICATION: THE KEY TO MEDICATION THERAPY SUCCESS

As new advances in medication therapy continue to evolve, it is imperative for pharmacists to build a strong pharmacist–patient relationship to ensure that optimal health outcomes are obtained for each patient. A key component in this relationship is effective communication. It is essential for student pharmacists to learn successful communication skills to gain an understanding of patient needs and in turn help patients in the most opportune way. This text does an excellent job of melding both theory and active-learning strategies to help student pharmacists learn to be adroit communicators.

The authors of this text, Drs. Min Liu and Lakesha Butler, are passionate about helping students become accomplished communicators. They exemplify the tenets of good communication in the classroom and in practice every day. The authors have written this text with the underlying philosophy that the application of theory through exercises and role-playing serves as a powerful tool for student pharmacists to work toward mastering the many nuances of communication. This learning-through-practice approach sets this text apart from others on communication.

This text is well organized into four sections and offers student pharmacists exposure to an excellent array of germane topics related to pharmacist–patient communication. After setting the stage with an overview section, the patient-centered aspects of communication are presented as the cornerstone of adherence to medication therapy. Given the changing demographics of the country, the section that addresses the needs of special patient populations (e.g., geriatric, pediatric, patients with low health literacy) is both timely and pertinent. The section on barriers and challenges to communication also emphasizes communication with other health professionals.

In summary, this text provides a solid foundation for student pharmacists to learn and practice their patient-centered communication skills. I am certain that the topics presented in this text will be valuable to the preparation of student pharmacists as catalysts in improving medication therapy for patients when they enter pharmacy practice.

Gireesh V. Gupchup, PhD, FAPhA
Dean and Professor
School of Pharmacy
Southern Illinois University Edwardsville

PREFACE

Welcome to *Patient Communication for Pharmacy*! As the authors of this text, we would like to congratulate you on taking this very important step toward building communication competency, which we believe is a highly necessary skill for pharmacists. Every day that you interact with patients, colleagues, and other healthcare providers, you are essentially using communication to positively influence someone's life. In this Preface, we hope to orient you toward the key features of this text in order to prepare you for this very exciting journey towards becoming more competent in your communication.

A COMMUNICATION SKILLS APPROACH

We believe that an abstract understanding of communication can be taught through principles and theories, but applicable communication skills must be learned through practice, reflection, and repetition. This text provides chapters that mesh theory, principles, and application all in one. Each chapter provides an introduction to important patient communication topics with theory and principles, followed by the opportunity for students to develop applicable communication skills through real patient case scenarios. By focusing on communication skills, we hope to help students understand not only the *what* and *why* of patient communication, but also provide them with the opportunity to learn the *how* of using communication to improve patient care.

A FOCUS ON PATIENT-CENTERED CARE

Patient-centered care is illustrated throughout this book. The American Pharmacists Association (APhA) defines *pharmaceutical care* as "a patient-centered, outcomes-oriented pharmacy practice that requires the pharmacist to work in concert with the patient and the patient's other healthcare providers" (n.d., p.1). It further identifies five practices that are key to delivering patient-centered care, including:

1) data collection,
2) information evaluation,
3) formulating a plan,
4) implementing the plan,
5) monitoring and modifying the plan and assuring positive outcome.

The success of each practice depends on the pharmacist's communication. Practices 1 and 4, for example, revolve mostly around the patient and quality communication is of the utmost importance. When formulating a plan or modifying it, the pharmacist should work with other healthcare providers as well as communicate the plan effectively to patients.

The pharmacy profession has fully embraced its departure from the dispensing role to one of patient-centered care at its core, and communication is a must-have tool for pharmacists in order to fulfill this role. While pharmacists may find themselves communicating in different contexts—including in small groups, to a general public, or via different media outlets—this text focuses primarily on the interpersonal communication dynamics between pharmacists and their patients. Successful communication is the only way to understand one's patients, win their trust, engage them in self-care behavior, and ultimately achieve patient care goals.

A Model of Repetition Through The LEARN, PRACTICE, and ASSESS Case Approaches

The LEARN, PRACTICE, and ASSESS patient cases at the end of each chapter are designed to help students hone communication skills through repetition.

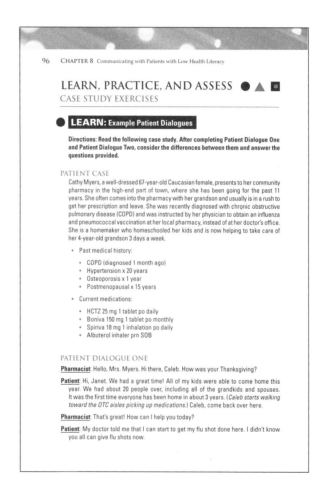

LEARN, PRACTICE, AND ASSESS ● ▲ ■
CASE STUDY EXERCISES

● LEARN: Example Patient Dialogues

Directions: Read the following case study. After completing Patient Dialogue One and Patient Dialogue Two, consider the differences between them and answer the questions provided.

PATIENT CASE
Cathy Myers, a well-dressed 67-year-old Caucasian female, presents to her community pharmacy in the high-end part of town, where she has been going for the past 11 years. She often comes into the pharmacy with her grandson and usually is in a rush to get her prescription and leave. She was recently diagnosed with chronic obstructive pulmonary disease (COPD) and was instructed by her physician to obtain an influenza and pneumococcal vaccination at her local pharmacy, instead of at her doctor's office. She is a homemaker who homeschooled her kids and is now helping to take care of her 4-year-old grandson 3 days a week.

- Past medical history:

  - COPD (diagnosed 1 month ago)
  - Hypertension x 20 years
  - Osteoporosis x 1 year
  - Postmenopausal x 15 years

- Current medications:

  - HCTZ 25 mg 1 tablet po daily
  - Boniva 150 mg 1 tablet po monthly
  - Spiriva 18 mg 1 inhalation po daily
  - Albuterol inhaler prn SOB

PATIENT DIALOGUE ONE

Pharmacist: Hello, Mrs. Myers. Hi there, Caleb. How was your Thanksgiving?

Patient: Hi, Janet. We had a great time! All of my kids were able to come home this year. We had about 20 people over, including all of the grandkids and spouses. It was the first time everyone has been home in about 3 years. (*Caleb starts walking toward the OTC aisles picking up medications.*) Caleb, come back over here.

Pharmacist: That's great! How can I help you today?

Patient: My doctor told me that I can start to get my flu shot done here. I didn't know you all can give flu shots now.

The LEARN section includes a patient case and two patient dialogue scenarios, one that features an ineffective patient dialogue related to the case, followed by an improved, more appropriate communication during the pharmacist–patient interactions. Instructors can use the discussion questions to invoke class discussion on the differences between the two dialogues and to help students make the connection between concepts in the chapters and the dialogues, while observing how patient communication makes a difference in patient outcomes.

x

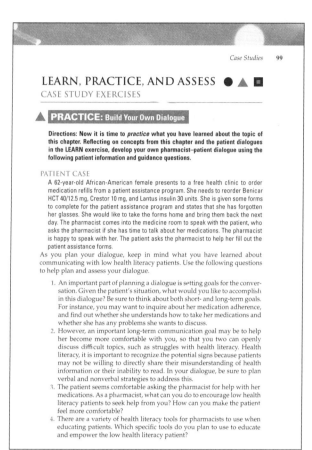

LEARN, PRACTICE, AND ASSESS ● ▲ ■
CASE STUDY EXERCISES

▲ PRACTICE: Build Your Own Dialogue

Directions: Now it is time to *practice* what you have learned about the topic of this chapter. Reflecting on concepts from this chapter and the patient dialogues in the LEARN exercise, develop your own pharmacist–patient dialogue using the following patient information and guidance questions.

PATIENT CASE

A 62-year-old African-American female presents to a free health clinic to order medication refills from a patient assistance program. She needs to reorder Benicar HCT 40/12.5 mg, Crestor 10 mg, and Lantus insulin 30 units. She is given some forms to complete for the patient assistance program and states that she has forgotten her glasses. She would like to take the forms home and bring them back the next day. The pharmacist comes into the medicine room to speak with the patient, who asks the pharmacist if she has time to talk about her medications. The pharmacist is happy to speak with her. The patient asks the pharmacist to help her fill out the patient assistance forms.

As you plan your dialogue, keep in mind what you have learned about communicating with low health literacy patients. Use the following questions to help plan and assess your dialogue.

1. An important part of planning a dialogue is setting goals for the conversation. Given the patient's situation, what would you like to accomplish in this dialogue? Be sure to think about both short- and long-term goals. For instance, you may want to inquire about her medication adherence, and find out whether she understands how to take her medications and whether she has any problems she wants to discuss.
2. However, an important long-term communication goal may be to help her become more comfortable with you, so that you two can openly discuss difficult topics, such as struggles with health literacy. Health literacy, it is important to recognize the potential signs because patients may not be willing to directly share their misunderstanding of health information or their inability to read. In your dialogue, be sure to plan verbal and nonverbal strategies to address this.
3. The patient seems comfortable asking the pharmacist for help with her medications. As a pharmacist, what can you do to encourage low health literacy patients to seek help from you? How can you make the patient feel more comfortable?
4. There are a variety of health literacy tools for pharmacists to use when educating patients. Which specific tools do you plan to use to educate and empower the low health literacy patient?

In the PRACTICE section, students apply what they have learned from the chapters and the LEARN dialogues by developing their own patient communication dialogue based on a provided patient case scenario. In this section, students are provided a set of guidance questions to ensure that they address key communication challenges and needs while designing the dialogue. Students transition from learning abstract concepts through observation to developing communication skills through guided application. Students can develop the PRACTICE dialogues in pairs or teams, and if possible, instructors should invite some students to role-play their dialogues. This can help facilitate a class discussion about the differences among the dialogues, and about the dynamic nature of pharmacy-patient communication.

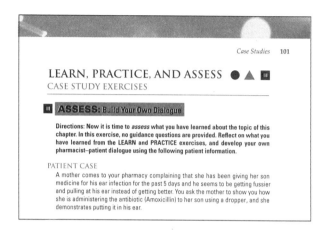

LEARN, PRACTICE, AND ASSESS ● ▲ ▣
CASE STUDY EXERCISES

▣ **ASSESS: Build Your Own Dialogue**

Directions: Now it is time to *assess* what you have learned about the topic of this chapter. In this exercise, no guidance questions are provided. Reflect on what you have learned from the LEARN and PRACTICE exercises, and develop your own pharmacist–patient dialogue using the following patient information.

PATIENT CASE
A mother comes to your pharmacy complaining that she has been giving her son medicine for his ear infection for the past 5 days and he seems to be getting fussier and pulling at his ear instead of getting better. You ask the mother to show you how she is administering the antibiotic (Amoxicillin) to her son using a dropper, and she demonstrates putting it in his ear.

The ASSESS section includes a final patient case scenario, and students are asked to create a communication dialogue based on what they have learned so far in the chapter. This section is designed to mimic real-life patient encounters, in which a pharmacist quickly gauges a patient's needs and responds with the appropriate communication strategies. Instructors can use this section to assess what students have learned in the chapter and whether they can translate what they have learned into actual patient care behavior. Through this repetition of practice and reflection, we believe the students can hone their communication skills in an expedient manner.

ADDITIONAL KEY FEATURES

Key terms are clearly defined in the text where the term first appears to help enhance comprehension and expand students' professional vocabulary.

End of Chapter Discussion Questions are intended to facilitate individual reflections or class discussions of each chapter's materials after students have completed the reading and the LEARN PRACTICE ASSESS exercises. Instructors can use these questions when they assign reflective essays, or to facilitate further discussion in certain areas of patient communication.

FOR THE INSTRUCTOR

The **Test Bank** includes true/false questions and multiple-choice questions of varying difficulty levels to assess student learning. Instructors can use the questions to test the student's recall of key information from the chapter, as well as assess their ability to apply these concepts in hypothetical scenarios.

Web Links of YouTube Videos provide two to three YouTube links that help illustrate concepts addressed in each chapter. A brief description of each video's content, source, and its connection to the course concepts is included to help instructors navigate this resource.

Slides in PowerPoint format for each chapter provide a starting template of key concepts to discuss during class lectures.

REVIEWERS

Christian B. Albano, PhD, MBA, MPH
Associate Professor
Concordia University Wisconsin

Dean L. Arneson, PharmD, PhD
Dean, School of Pharmacy
Concodia University

Peter M. Brody, Jr., BS, PharmD
Clinical Assistant Professor
SUNY at Buffalo School of Pharmacy and Pharmaceutical Sciences

Bonnie Brown, PharmD
Associate Professor
Butler University College of Pharmacy and Health Sciences

Sherrill J. Brown, DVM, PharmD, BCPS
University of Montana Skaggs School of Pharmacy

Chris Gillette, PhD
Assistant Professor & Director, Simulated Learning Experiences
Marshal University School of Pharmacy

Kristen Pate, PharmD, BCACP
University of Louisiana at Monroe College of Pharmacy

Elizabeth Perry, PharmD, BCPS
Assistant Professor
ULM College of Pharmacy

REFERENCE

American Pharmacists Association (n.d.). *Principles of practice for pharmaceutical care.* Retrieved from http://www.pharmacist.com/principles-practice-pharmaceutical-care

PART I

OVERVIEW

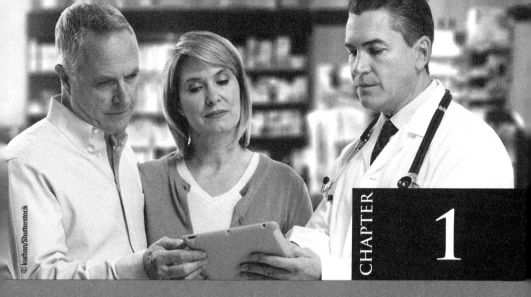

© kurhan/Shutterstock

CHAPTER 1

PHARMACY PATIENT COMMUNICATION: A TRANSACTIONAL MODEL

LEARNING OBJECTIVES

At the end of this chapter, students should be able to:

- Explain the Transactional Model and its key assumptions.
- Explain communication as driven by instrumental and relational goals.
- Define competent communication and its key elements.
- Articulate the role of ethics in pharmacist–patient communication.
- Generate communication strategies to engage the patient as a partner in a therapeutic relationship.

KEY TERMS

Communication competence

Instrumental goals

Knowledge

Motivation

Relational goals

Skill

Think back to a recent encounter you had with another person, whether it was communication for personal or professional purposes. What messages were communicated? How were those messages transmitted? Was anything happening in the background, and if so, how did it affect your communication with the other person? Did the communication fulfill your needs or goals? What about the needs or goals of the other person? What relationship, if any, did the two of you have prior to the interaction, and in what ways might the relationship have changed after the interaction? Questions like these remind us that communication is complicated and shaped by a multitude of factors. To communicate effectively, one must first understand the elements of a typical communication encounter between two individuals.

ELEMENTS OF THE TRANSACTIONAL MODEL

Communication scholars developed a Transactional Model of communication to help us understand the following basic elements that exist in communication encounters:

- The communication situation
- The environment
- The sender(s) and receiver(s)
- The message(s)
- The communication channel(s)
- The feedback
- The noise, also known as the communication barrier(s)

Figure 1-1 illustrates this model.

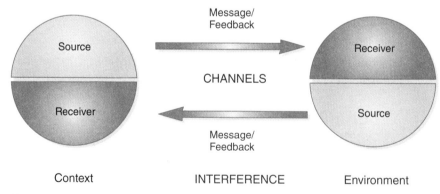

Figure 1-1   Transactional Model of Communication.

Understanding the different elements of communication as a transactional process can help us diagnose problematic communication exchanges and strategize and maximize our communication effectiveness. Read the following example scenarios, and consider which element(s) of the Transactional Model may be most important in each scenario:

- A patient arrives to pick up a new prescription indicated for depression. The pharmacist asks the patient if he has any questions or concerns about the medication. The patient says yes but stops himself mid-sentence, after noticing the line of people waiting behind him.
- The pharmacist wants to call a physician's office about a prescription refill. Because the patient has complained of some side effects, he wants to share those concerns with the physician and recommend a new medication that might work better. The pharmacist thinks about how to approach the physician, who is known to be impatient about this kind of conversation.
- A pharmacist meets a deaf patient for the first time in her career. She decides to educate herself about how to best communicate with deaf patients. She considers different options, including print materials, visuals, or the use of interpreting services.

Many of the chapters in this text focus on how to best communicate with specific patient populations, given a certain characteristic of the population such as age or language skills (i.e., a focus on *sender/receiver*). Some chapters focus on topics that may be particularly challenging to communicate about, including sensitive topics or emotionally charged conversations (i.e., a focus on *message*). We also discuss how the different professional contexts in which a pharmacist's practices may influence patient communication (i.e., a focus on *context*), how different barriers may result in less effective communication (i.e., a focus on *noise* or *barrier*), and how new communication techniques hold the potential for more efficient patient communication (i.e., a focus on *communication channel*). We encourage you to apply the Transactional Model and its different elements to the rest of this text, especially when completing the LEARN, PRACTICE, and ASSESS exercises.

KEY ASSUMPTIONS OF THE TRANSACTIONAL MODEL

A key difference between the Transactional Model and the earlier models of communication is that it accounts for the *simultaneous sending and receiving of messages* by all parties involved. When a patient explains to you her concerns about a medication, she sends you verbal messages, which you try to comprehend while taking note of her tone of voice, facial expressions, and other nonverbal cues. At the same time, the patient is likely also aware of and responsive to your body language and eye contact. When interacting with a patient or colleague, remember that all parties, regardless of who is talking, are sending verbal and nonverbal messages and collaboratively contribute to the interaction.

Following the previous assumption, the model also assumes that communicators in a conversation *share the credit* when communication is effective and mutually satisfying and should *share the blame* when communication breakdown, conflict, or other undesirable outcomes occur. At times, this is easier said than done. We have likely all heard someone say that "We had a fight, but it was not my fault," or that "He is always so rude, which is why I do not try to be nice to him." Communication is both a science and a form of art. It can be difficult, if at all possible, to definitively establish "what caused what" or "who is responsible for what" with regard to communication processes and outcomes. The most fruitful thing to do is to recognize communication as a two-way street, as suggested by the Transactional Model, and to be mindful of the various elements that shape our communication experience.

Another assumption of the Transactional Model is that *communication is essential to building and maintaining relationships*. As a pharmacist, maintaining a good relationship with colleagues, other healthcare professionals, and patients and their caretakers benefits your patients by improving patient care, but it also provides you with such benefits as a better work environment and higher job satisfaction. For example, humor, empathy, and active listening are communication tools useful for improving relationship outcomes. *Humor* can lighten the mood of the conversation and helps build a sense of closeness. *Empathy* requires the ability to recognize the emotional state and needs of the other person so that you can try to feel what the person might be feeling. This important communication tool will be discussed in more detail in the chapter on Empathy and Patient Communication. *Active listening* is the act of mindfully concentrating on what is being said to improve comprehension, which is very helpful for building rapport. Fundamentally, these are all communication tools. Hence, some people argue that communication is the most important tool for building and maintaining personal or professional relationships. The Transactional Model of communication recognizes the central role communication plays in shaping our relationship outcomes.

GOALS AND IDEALS FOR PHARMACIST–PATIENT COMMUNICATION

Although not highlighted in the Transactional Model, we would like you to think of communication as a goal-driven act. Granted, as you greet a colleague in the morning, or speak to a patient on the phone, you likely are not consciously thinking about specific goals you would like to accomplish with each act. Nonetheless, our communication is driven by goals that we need and/or want to accomplish. Goals can be **instrumental** (McCornack, 2009); for instance, you may need to explain to a parent how to give her child asthma treatment for the first time, or convince a colleague to do you a favor. Instrumental goals are specific things you would like to accomplish with your communication. Goals can also be **relational**; for instance, we may strategically communicate in a certain way to establish, maintain, improve, change, or at times terminate relationships. We greet someone with a "How have you been?" not because we want an update on the person's recent life events (which would be an instrumental goal) but because it is a friendly conversation opener and socially expected. As we engage in daily communication, it is helpful to think about goals important to us and to the other communicators.

How should we define *good communication*? Is it ideal for communication to have all of our goals accomplished because we consider it a goal-driven act? What about the goals of others? What about situations where various goals clash with one another? For instance, what if accomplishing an instrumental goal (e.g., finishing up with your patients as fast as you can) requires sacrificing a relational goal (i.e., making a new patient feel more comfortable with you)? What would be the *competent* thing to do?

UNDERSTANDING COMPETENT COMMUNICATION

Communication competence is the ability to choose a communication behavior that is appropriate, effective, and ethical for a given situation (McCornack, 2009). Ideally, our communication is *effective* in helping us accomplish goals, *appropriate* for the situation given the relationship and context, and *ethical* in being truthful, respectful, and inclusive. Again, one can easily think of scenarios in which all three cannot be accomplished. In this text, we focus primarily on how to be *effective* when communicating with different patients and how to adapt our communication strategies so that they are *appropriate* to unique patient needs and situations. It is, however, of the utmost importance to always keep in mind key ethical principles and professional guidelines to ensure that our communications meet the highest possible ethical standards. See the next section on Ethics and Pharmacists for a discussion on ethical principles applicable to pharmacy professionals.

The model most often used to describe communication competence was proposed by Spitzberg and Cupach (1984) and includes three components: (1) knowledge, (2) skill, and (3) motivation. See **Figure 1-2** for an adaptation of this model for the purposes of this text.

As you can see, the **Knowledge** category determines whether cognitively we can understand the communication dynamics and strategize which behavior is best suited for a given situation. The **Skill** category determines whether we have the ability and tools to enact the behavior in the given context. The **Motivation** category, shaped by our desires, interests, and values, ultimately determines whether we have the willpower to enhance our knowledge and improve our skills. Active listening, for instance, is a skill and takes effort and practice. Another useful communication skill is asking open-ended questions to gain a more complete understanding of the patient. These skills are often underutilized because they take effort and

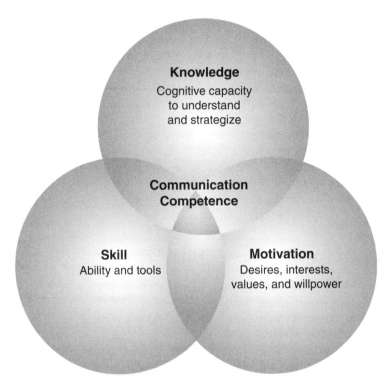

Figure 1-2 Model of Communication Competence.

time. Only when pharmacy professionals have the right knowledge and motivation will such communication skills likely be used. As you can see, to develop communication competency, one must work on all three fronts.

By reading a text dedicated to pharmacy patient communication, you have indicated that you value patient communication as an important tool for pharmacists. We congratulate you for having the *motivation* to become a competent communicator; *knowledge* and *skills* of communication can be learned. Chances are that none of us will be able to say one day that we have perfected the skills of communication. Instead, let us all commit ourselves to a lifelong journey to improving our communication skills!

ETHICS AND PHARMACISTS

The American Pharmacists Association (APhA) adopted its Code of Ethics in 1994 (APhA, 2015). In 2007, the American Association of Colleges of Pharmacy approved a revised Oath of a Pharmacist. These are key ethical guidelines for the pharmacy profession.

In addition, when communicating to or about a patient, patient confidentiality is not only a professional and ethical requirement, it is also

AMERICAN PHARMACISTS ASSOCIATION'S CODE OF ETHICS FOR PHARMACISTS

Preamble: Pharmacists are health professionals who assist individuals in making the best use of medications. This Code, prepared and supported by pharmacists, is intended to state publicly the principles that form the fundamental basis of the roles and responsibilities of pharmacists. These principles, based on moral obligations and virtues, are established to guide pharmacists in relationships with patients, health professionals, and society.

I.   A pharmacist respects the covenantal relationship between the patient and pharmacist.

II. A pharmacist promotes the good of every patient in a caring, compassionate, and confidential manner.

III. A pharmacist respects the autonomy and dignity of each patient.

IV. A pharmacist acts with honesty and integrity in professional relationships.

V.   A pharmacist maintains professional competence.

VI. A pharmacist respects the values and abilities of colleagues and other health professionals.

VII. A pharmacist serves individual, community, and societal needs.

VIII. A pharmacist seeks justice in the distribution of health resources.

AMERICAN ASSOCIATION OF COLLEGES OF PHARMACY'S OATH OF A PHARMACIST

"I promise to devote myself to a lifetime of service to others through the profession of pharmacy. In fulfilling this vow:

- I will consider the welfare of humanity and relief of suffering my primary concerns.
- I will apply my knowledge, experience, and skills to the best of my ability to assure optimal outcomes for my patients.
- I will respect and protect all personal and health information entrusted to me.
- I will accept the lifelong obligation to improve my professional knowledge and competence.
- I will hold myself and my colleagues to the highest principles of our profession's moral, ethical, and legal conduct.
- I will embrace and advocate changes that improve patient care.
- I will utilize my knowledge, skills, experiences, and values to prepare the next generation of pharmacists.

I take these vows voluntarily with the full realization of the responsibility with which I am entrusted by the public."

required by law. The Health Insurance Portability and Accountability Act (HIPAA) was signed into law in 1996 to address patient privacy, specifically referring to personal patient data known as protected health information (PHI) (U.S. Department of Health and Human Services, n.d.). PHI includes specific personal information pertaining to every patient, such as their name, date of birth, and social security number. This information can be provided in three primary forms: written, electronic, and oral. For example, pharmacy records and electronic medical records are PHI and must be protected and kept confidential. Failure to do so could result in punishment ranging from a fine to imprisonment. When a patient is under the care of a healthcare professional, the patient's medical information cannot be discussed with anyone else unless the patient allows it. However, there are some exceptions to PHI that may vary from state to state, including suspected abuse and certain contagious diseases. As a healthcare professional, it is your responsibility to protect your patient's health information through all modes of communication.

DISCUSSION QUESTIONS

1. As you read the lists of ethical guidelines, which ones are more or less applicable to you?
2. The APhA adopted its Code of Ethics in 1994. The practice and discipline of pharmacy has seen significant changes since then. In what ways do you think the Code of Ethics can be updated?
3. Among the ethical guidelines, are there any that are particularly relevant to patient communication and interaction? Please explain.
4. As discussed in this text, communication is a goal-driven act. When a patient's goal conflicts with the pharmacist's goal, what would be the appropriate and ethical thing for the pharmacist to do?

REFERENCES

American Association of Colleges of Pharmacy. (2007). *Oath of a pharmacist.* Retrieved from http://www.pharmacist.com/oath-pharmacist

American Pharmacists Association. (2015). *Code of ethics for pharmacists.* Retrieved from http://www.pharmacist.com/code-ethics

McCornack, S. (2009). *Reflect and relate: An introduction to interpersonal communication* (2nd ed.). Boston, MA: Bedford/St. Martin's.

Spitzberg, B. H., & Cupach, W. R. (1984). *Interpersonal communication competence.* Beverly Hills, CA: Sage.

U.S. Department of Health and Human Services. (n.d.). *Health information privacy.* Retrieved from http://www.hhs.gov/ocr/privacy/index.html

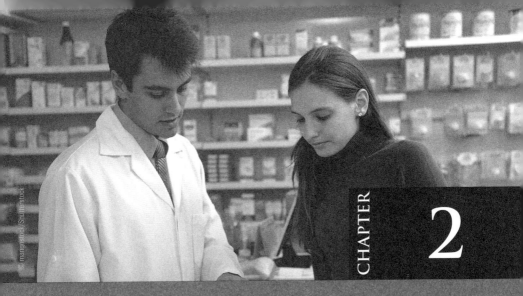

CHAPTER 2

PHARMACIST–PATIENT RELATIONSHIP: A COLLABORATIVE APPROACH

LEARNING OBJECTIVES

At the end of this chapter, students should be able to:

- ▸ Define *patient empowerment*.
- ▸ Articulate the importance of understanding and negotiating expectations of patients and pharmacists.
- ▸ Use the concept of control to differentiate among modes of pharmacist–patient relationships.
- ▸ Generate communication strategies to engage patients as partners in a therapeutic relationship.

KEY TERMS

Collaborative relationship

Consumerist relationship

Paternalistic relationship

Patient empowerment

Unengaged relationship

The relationship between pharmacists and their patients has been conceptualized in different ways. The pharmacy profession has evolved from its early dispensing role to include responsibilities of patient education, patient advocacy, and medication management, to name a few (Lai, Trac, & Lovett, 2013). With these additional responsibilities, the pharmacist–patient relationship is being redefined. What relationship do you wish to have with your patients? What relationship do you think your patients wish to have with you? More importantly, what relationship will lead to the best health outcomes for the patient?

PATIENT EMPOWERMENT

Healthcare professions have embraced the concept of patient empowerment as an essential component in achieving the ideal patient–provider relationship. **Patient empowerment** is defined as helping patients discover and develop the inherent capacity to be responsible for one's own life (Funnell & Anderson, 2003). The premise is that while healthcare providers, including pharmacists, may be experts of medical conditions and development of treatment plans, patients are experts of their own illness experiences; only when both sets of expertise are combined can the optimum patient outcomes be achieved. This is an important shift from the paternalistic paradigm where patients were to be obedient and follow providers' orders, a shift that might be difficult for both parties involved. Patients and healthcare professionals must understand the need to see patients as part of the healthcare team to ensure quality of care and to decrease medication errors.

However, it is important to recognize in any relationship, whether personal or professional, that the roles and responsibilities are negotiated by all parties involved. Pharmacists come to patient encounters with expectations for which patient care and relationship outcomes they want to achieve. It is important to recognize that patients also come with expectations, which are likely shaped by a variety of factors including their previous interactions with pharmacists, their experiences with other healthcare professionals, their healthcare needs, and other sociocultural factors such as education and socioeconomic status. The key is to ensure that the pharmacist–patient relationship reflects the expectations of both parties. In a 2007 study of 500 patients and 500 pharmacists conducted by Worley and colleagues, they concluded that when pharmacists and their patients agree on the relationship roles of both parties, both the relationship and patient care outcomes are optimized.

As we consider the importance of patient empowerment, pharmacists must understand the unique needs and expectations of each patient. Instead of a one-size-fits-all approach to patient empowerment, consider the following questions for each patient:

- Given the unique health needs of this patient, what level of empowerment and patient involvement is ideal?

- Will the patient benefit from playing a more active role in his or her care? Is this patient ready to become more involved?
- Which barriers exist that prevent this patient from taking a more active role in his or her health care?
- As a pharmacist, what is the best way for me to enable this patient to become a more educated and involved party in his or her healthcare outcomes?

A COLLABORATIVE APPROACH

It has been argued that any provider–patient relationship can be understood from a perspective of control (Kelner, 2000). **Table 2-1** describes four modes of the patient–provider relationship, which differ in how much control the two parties have in the relationship (Greenfield, 2001). In a relationship with high provider control and low patient control, known as a **paternalistic relationship**, the provider is dominant and decides what he or she believes to be in the patient's best interest while the patient assumes a more passive role. In the less likely scenario of high patient control and low provider control, referred to as a **consumerist relationship**, the provider adopts a fairly passive role, acceding to the requests of an actively engaged patient—for example, the patient may request a change in medication or the ordering of a specific lab. The general consensus is that the **unengaged relationship** of low provider control and low patient control is not conducive to informed decision making by the patient. However, a **collaborative relationship**, one of high provider control and high patient control, closely resembles the concept of patient empowerment and is believed to be ideal for ensuring a truly collaborative relationship between the provider and the patient.

Table 2-1: Four Modes of the Patient–Provider Relationship		
	High Patient Control	**Low Patient Control**
High Provider Control	Collaborative relationship	Paternalistic relationship
Low Provider Control	Consumerist relationship	Default/unengaged relationship

Every patient encounter offers an opportunity for understanding patient needs and expectations and for negotiating the ideal level of patient empowerment. For instance, in the following scenarios, the patient needs and expectations are all different, each with unique patient care requirements. It is important for a pharmacist to take a truly *patient-centered approach* with each patient and negotiate a pharmacist–patient relationship that is most beneficial to the specific patient.

- A single parent in her early 20s whose 2-year-old child is being put on asthma medication for the first time.
- A diabetes patient who has been diligent in taking her daily oral medications is devastated to learn that she has to start taking insulin. Patients typically think that insulin is the last-resort treatment for diabetes.
- A hospice patient who is on several medications for pain control.
- A patient in his 50s who has been on a medication for his heart condition for almost 10 years and is now starting a new medication; the doctor also wants the patient to make changes to his diet and to exercise more.
- A LEP (limited English proficiency) patient is on antibiotics for 10 days for a respiratory infection; it is unclear how much the patient understands about her condition.

In a feature story published in *Academic Pharmacy Now*, the Medication Therapy Management Clinic operated by the University of Chicago College of Pharmacy uses a patient empowerment approach to counsel a diverse patient population on how to handle multiple medications (American Association of Colleges of Pharmacy, 2008). The program's goal is to enable patients to play an essential part in their own care rather than taking that role away from them. This is key to building a collaborative relationship with patients. Patients will always present with unique needs and challenges when it comes to understanding their conditions and managing their medications. A truly collaborative approach to building relationships with patients will allow pharmacists to better understand each and every one of their patients and respond to their unique needs and challenges.

LEARN, PRACTICE, AND ASSESS
CASE STUDY EXERCISES

● **LEARN: Example Patient Dialogues**

Directions: Read the following case study. After completing Patient Dialogue One and Patient Dialogue Two, consider the differences between them and answer the questions provided.

PATIENT CASE

A 49-year-old female who has had diabetes for the last 8 years has been taking her oral diabetes medications daily with minimal missed doses. She visits her endocrinologist for a follow up and is discouraged by the current uncontrolled state of her diabetes, despite taking her medications and "cutting back" on her meal portions. She is maxed out on the oral medications and is told by her doctor that she has to start insulin today to get her diabetes under control.

- Current HgA1C = 9% (goal = less than 7%)

She is referred to the pharmacist for education on insulin injection, and the patient shows both verbal and nonverbal cues of nervousness (minimal eye contact, wringing of hands, and consistent use of "um's" when talking).

PATIENT DIALOGUE ONE

Pharmacist: Hello, Ms. Todd. I am the clinical pharmacist, and your doctor wants me to discuss with you how to start and adjust your insulin.

Patient: (*The patient has minimal eye contact with the pharmacist and wrings her hands.*) Um, okay.

Pharmacist: You can inject insulin into three different places: your stomach, your buttock, or the back of your arm. You should choose just one part of the body because each place absorbs the insulin at different rates. I recommend that you inject into your stomach. You should rotate sites on the stomach each time you inject. You will be starting Lantus 10 units and will inject at night before going to bed and . . . (*As the pharmacist is talking, the patient starts sweating and continues fidgeting more in her chair.*)

Patient: (*The patient interrupts the pharmacist.*) Um, will this hurt?

Pharmacist: It will hurt a little, but you will get used to it, and it will help to better control your diabetes. You should pinch up the fat on your stomach and inject 10 units directly into this area (*demonstrating to patient using a ball*) and hold for 10 seconds to allow all of the insulin to go into the stomach. You will increase by 3 units every other day until your fasting blood sugar is 100–130. Do you have any questions?

Patient: Um, I really do not want to start taking insulin.

Pharmacist: It will be okay. There are many people on insulin and, like I said before, it will help better control your diabetes. I will call you this week to see how it is going.

Patient: Um, okay (*still wringing hands, visibly nervous*).

(One week later the pharmacist calls the patient to inquire about insulin use and blood sugar readings, and the patient states that she did not start insulin.)

PATIENT DIALOGUE TWO

Pharmacist: Hello, Ms. Todd. I am the clinical pharmacist, and your doctor wants me to discuss with you how to start and adjust your insulin.

Patient: (*The patient has minimal eye contact with the pharmacist and wrings her hands.*) Um, okay.

Pharmacist: (*Looks up and sees the patient's body language.*) Ms. Todd, you seem a bit worried to me. Can you share your concerns?

Patient: (*Looks up at the pharmacist.*) Well, to be honest, I am really nervous about starting insulin.

Pharmacist: That is a normal feeling, and I want to help you feel more comfortable. What concerns you about starting insulin?

Patient: I am afraid of needles; the idea of having to inject myself every day is just too much. Also, it wasn't supposed to get this bad. I guess I am frustrated that my diabetes has gotten to this point because I have been taking my medications every day and changed my diet! (*Frustrated and deflated.*)

Pharmacist: I understand your frustration, and you should be commended for all of your efforts. I want to clear up the misunderstanding about being at a bad point in your diabetes control. Many people think that if you have to start insulin then your diabetes is bad, but that couldn't be further from the truth. Insulin should actually be used sooner rather than later to help control your diabetes better. This is going to be a great and effective step in getting your diabetes under control. My uncle has had diabetes for 20 years, and I remember him feeling the same way you do when he had to be put on insulin. But once he conquered his fears and started taking the insulin as prescribed, he told me how much better he felt: He had more energy, his eyesight improved, and above all, his blood sugar was the best it had ever been. Are these goals that you want to achieve?

Patient: Yes, I would love to have more energy and have my blood sugars where they need to be. I guess since you put it that way, this would be best for me, but how do I inject myself? Will you help me?

Pharmacist: Of course, that's what I am here for. I will walk you through the entire process and follow up with you by phone in a week to help you. I also would like to meet with you at least once a month to provide more diabetes education and address any concerns and questions you may have. We also have monthly diabetes group meetings that you can attend that discuss everything there is to know about diabetes and insulin. I am here to work with you and your doctor to help better control your diabetes. It is important that we work *together* to accomplish the goal of improved diabetes control and prevention of complications. Are you ready to get your diabetes under control?

Patient: Yes, I am! Thank you so much for helping me to put things into perspective. I guess a second of pain from the needle each day does not compare to possibly going blind, my kidneys failing, or losing a limb.

Pharmacist: Exactly, Ms. Todd. It's great to see that you are ready to take this under your control. What I've seen with my diabetes patients is that when the patient sticks to the treatment plan, diabetes really does not need to take over your life. If you run into any problems, please be sure to let us know and we'll be happy to help.

Patient: I really appreciate you taking the time to talk with me and offering to help me along the way. Thanks!

Discussion Questions for the **LEARN** Exercise

1. What key signs of apprehension were displayed by the patient during the first healthcare encounter?
2. Compare and discuss the perspectives of control displayed in the two patient dialogues.
3. How did the pharmacist empower the patient to start insulin in Dialogue Two?

LEARN, PRACTICE, AND ASSESS
CASE STUDY EXERCISES

 PRACTICE: Build Your Own Dialogue

Directions: Now it is time to *practice* what you have learned about the topic of this chapter. Reflecting on concepts from this chapter and the patient dialogues in the LEARN exercise, develop your own pharmacist–patient dialogue using the following patient information and guidance questions.

PATIENT CASE

A 22-year-old mother has an 18-month-old daughter with newly diagnosed asthma. The mother is not familiar with asthma and is unsure of how her daughter "caught" asthma. The child's pediatrician orders a nebulizer machine (an electric breathing machine usually for pediatric patients with asthma that compresses liquid medicine into an inhaled mist) for the child and sends prescriptions for albuterol solution to be used in the nebulizer. The mother presents to your pharmacy to pick up the albuterol but is very unsure of how to use the nebulizer machine and what she can do to help prevent her daughter from having an asthma attack. She is really frustrated.

As you plan your dialogue, keep in mind what you have learned about communicating with a collaborative approach. Use the following questions to help plan and assess your dialogue.

1. An important part of planning a dialogue is setting goals for the conversation. Given the situation, what would you like to accomplish in this dialogue? Be sure to think about both short- and long-term goals. For instance, you may want to initially dispel the mother's thought of the daughter catching asthma, provide education about the etiology of asthma, and discuss and demonstrate how to use a nebulizer machine. However, a more important goal is to communicate to the mother that you want to help her and her child and would like to listen to what she has to say.

2. It is important to recognize that patients come with expectations that are shaped by various factors. The patient is frustrated because no one has taken the time to educate her on the details of asthma and how to use a nebulizer. How will you address the mother's preconceived expectations during your dialogue?

3. Ensure that you are not displaying a paternalistic approach when communicating with the mother. How do you plan to involve the patient's mother as part of the healthcare team? What will be her specific role in managing her daughter's asthma?

4. Define *empowerment.* How will you empower the mother to take an active role in her daughter's health? What challenges might make it difficult for the mother to take more control of her child's health condition?
5. How will you ensure that the mother understands how to treat her daughter's asthma with both nonpharmacologic and pharmacologic treatments?

YOUR DIALOGUE HERE

LEARN, PRACTICE, AND ASSESS
CASE STUDY EXERCISES

☐ ASSESS: Build Your Own Dialogue

Directions: Now it is time to *assess* what you have learned about the topic of this chapter. In this exercise, no guidance questions are provided. Reflect on what you have learned from the LEARN and PRACTICE exercises, and develop your own pharmacist–patient dialogue using the following patient information.

PATIENT CASE

A 47-year-old truck driver was recently discharged from the hospital after being diagnosed with a pulmonary embolism. He smokes two packs of cigarettes per day and is in the contemplation stage of smoking cessation. He presents to the warfarin clinic for his initial visit and an INR check and warfarin dose adjustment by the pharmacist. The pharmacist wants the patient to understand the importance of taking an active role in his health by quitting smoking and taking his warfarin as prescribed. The patient is not completely motivated to quit smoking and is not clear on how his social history contributed to the pulmonary embolism. This is his first one-on-one interaction with a pharmacist.

YOUR DIALOGUE HERE

DISCUSSION QUESTIONS

1. Which techniques do you plan to use when educating patients who may need empowerment for their health care?
2. In your opinion or observation, are there any scenarios in which a paternalistic or consumerist approach to the patient–pharmacist relationship is better than a collaborative approach? Please explain.
3. Which patient or provider factors might make it difficult to maintain a truly collaborative relationship between a patient and a pharmacist?
4. Have you encountered cases in which patients could benefit from taking a more active role in their health care? What prevented the patients from taking a more empowered role then?

REFERENCES

American Association of Colleges of Pharmacy. (2008). Empowering patients through medication therapy management. *Academic Pharmacy Now, 1*(4). Retrieved from http://www.aacp.org/news/academicpharmnow/documents/jul%20aug%20 2008%20apn.pdf

Funnell, M. M., & Anderson, R. M. (2003). Patient empowerment: A look back, a look ahead. *The Diabetes Educator, 29*(3), 455–464.

Greenfield, J. A. (2001). Medical decisionmaking: Models of the doctor-patient relationship. *Healthcare Communication Review, 1*(1). Retrieved from http://www .healthcp.org /hcr/v1n1-medical-decisionmaking.pdf

Kelner, M. (2000). The therapeutic relationship under fire. In M. Kelner, B. Wellman, B. Pescosolido, & M. Saks, *Complementary and alternative medicine: Challenge and change* (pp. 79–98). Amsterdam, The Netherlands: Harwood.

Lai, E., Trac, L., & Lovett, A. (2013). Expanding the pharmacist's role in public health. *Universal Journal of Public Health, 1*(3), 79–85.

Worley, M. M., Schommer, J. C., Brown, L. M., Hadsall, R. S., Ranelli, P. L., Stratton, T. P., & Uden, D. L. (2007). Pharmacists' and patients' roles in the pharmacist-patient relationship: Are pharmacists and patients reading from the same relationship script? *Research in Social and Administrative Pharmacy, 3*(1), 47–69.

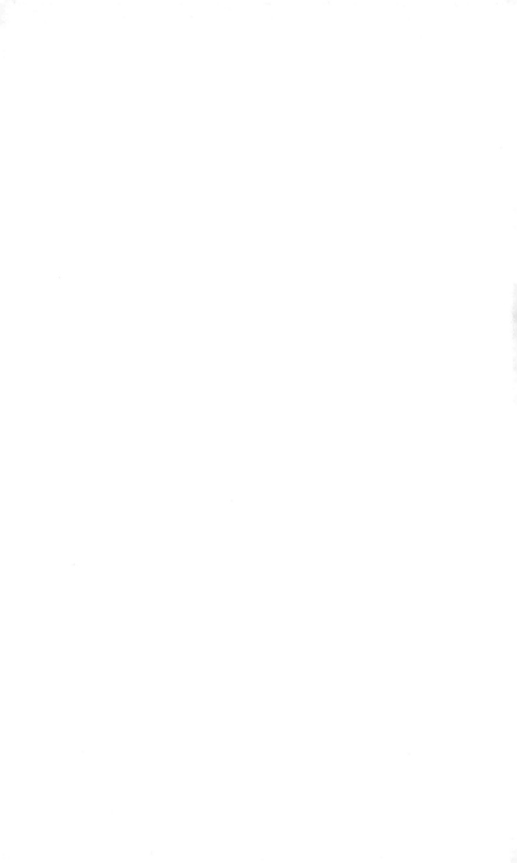

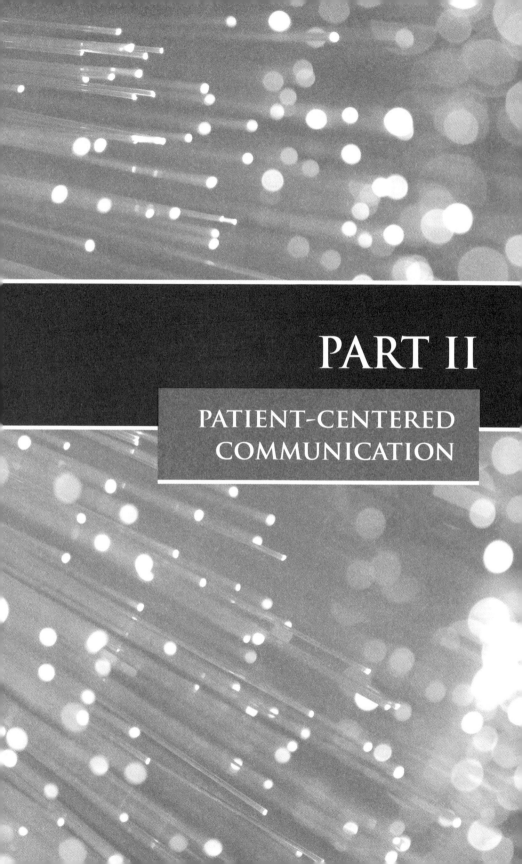

PART II

PATIENT-CENTERED
COMMUNICATION

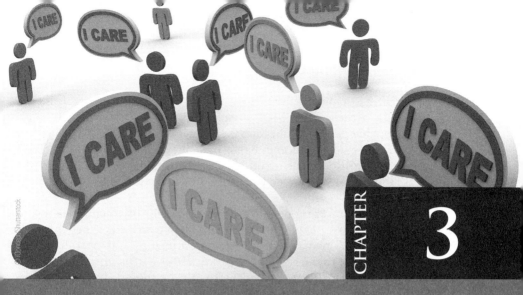

EMPATHY AND PATIENT COMMUNICATION

LEARNING OBJECTIVES

At the end of this chapter, students should be able to:

▸ Define *empathy* and explain its importance to pharmacist–patient communication.

▸ Identify verbal and nonverbal communication strategies to communicate empathy.

▸ Recognize barriers to communicating empathy.

▸ Generate communication strategies to assess patient needs and communicate empathy.

KEY TERMS

Clinical empathy

Cognitive empathy

Emotional empathy

Empathy

Most, if not all, students of pharmacy (as well as other healthcare professions) enter the field because they want to help people—they want to use their expertise to enable people to improve their health. Understandably, they feel frustrated at times when it seems like a patient simply does not want their help. As Theodore Roosevelt reminded us, "No one cares how much you know, until they know how much you care." To show your patients how much you care, empathy is essential.

Empathy is a vital component in the relationship between a healthcare provider and his or her patient. Empathy in patient care leads to better health outcomes, including increased medication compliance and overall higher patient satisfaction. Provider empathy is crucial for a satisfying relationship with patients. When patients are satisfied with the therapeutic relationship with their provider, the lines of communication become more open and honest. Patients are also more likely to listen and trust their provider.

WHAT IS EMPATHY?

In the context of the patient–healthcare provider relationship, **empathy** has been defined as the ability to understand the patient's experiences, pain, suffering, and perspective, as well as the ability to communicate this understanding and an intention to help (Nightingale, Yarnold, & Greenberg, 1991). In layperson's terms, empathy is putting yourself in someone else's shoes and understanding that person. There is an inherent communication dimension to empathy. Consider this: No matter how much you understand or care about your patient, if you fail to communicate your understanding and intention to help, the patient will not perceive you as having empathy.

Empathy is not the same as sympathy, and scholars in various healthcare fields have attempted to distinguish the two for theoretical and practical purposes. Sympathy, predominantly an affective attribute, is when you feel sorry for someone but do not feel the same emotions. Empathy, which has *cognitive and emotional* dimensions (Mercer & Reynolds, 2002), is placing yourself in that person's situation and responding based on either similar personal experience or through vicarious understanding. **Cognitive empathy** occurs when one makes a conscious effort to recognize and understand the other person's emotional state, often referred to as *perspective taking*. **Emotional empathy**, often referred to as *vicarious sharing of emotions*, occurs when we respond in a certain way, often subconsciously or unconsciously, to emotions displayed by others.

To empathize is to feel *with* the patient, whereas to sympathize is to feel *for* the patient. Empathy in health care involves an understanding of patients' concerns and the capacity to communicate this understanding and an intention to help. Sympathy, if excessive, may limit the provider's objectivity in caring for the patient. Empathy allows patients to feel as if you understand what they are going through.

HOW TO COMMUNICATE EMPATHY

In a study by Hojat and colleagues (2001), healthcare providers who practice in more people-oriented contexts such as primary care displayed more empathy toward patients than those in more technology-oriented contexts such as surgery. Because pharmacists mostly work directly with patients, empathy is an essential skill in order to serve their patients well. Empathy can be displayed verbally and nonverbally; here we review some techniques for communicating empathy.

Nonverbal cues of empathy include offering a more private setting for discussion, using a warm and caring tone of voice, maintaining direct eye contact (without being overbearing), nodding your head while listening, offering tissue if the person is crying, and leaning toward the patient. In a 2013 study by Montague, Chen, Xu, Chewning, and Barrett, patient participants rated clinicians who used more direct eye contact and social touch with them as more caring, having more empathy, and in general being more likeable. Empathy is most relevant when a patient is in distress. You should do whatever you can to communicate to the patient that "I am here and I would like to listen." The key to empathy is to communicate to patients that you want to understand their perspective and help address any concerns or issues they may have. Empathy helps you build rapport with the patient, which can set the tone of the interaction and allow the patient to feel comfortable with you. Another important nonverbal aspect of empathy is listening. When you are putting yourself in the patient's shoes, you must keep an open mind to listen in a nonjudgmental and supportive way.

We can also demonstrate empathy through our verbal responses. With the desire to help, you may be tempted to offer patients advice as to what you think they should do or how you think they should feel. Discussing what you would do if you were in the situation is not empathy; instead, you should allow patients to feel comfortable discussing how they feel and offer understanding while recognizing the uniqueness of their experience. According to Barrett-Lennard (1993), empathy is a communicative process that consists of three phases. Phase 1 is the inner process of empathetic listening, where the pharmacist listens to the patient actively and tries to understand the patient's perspective. In phase 2, the pharmacist attempts to convey empathetic understanding of the patient's experience. Phase 3 is the patient's awareness of and reflection on this exchange of thoughts and emotions. As a result of this empathy cycle, patients feel understood and comforted, and the reflective attitude enables them to better manage their emotions and possibly better cope with their situation. Some scholars believe that feeling comforted and being able to reflect are two key functions of empathy for patients during medical encounters (Lussier & Richard, 2007).

BARRIERS TO EMPATHY

While few would deny the benefits of empathy, it can be difficult to communicate with empathy given the many barriers that exist. Consider the following barriers that may limit a pharmacist's ability to communicate with a patient in an empathic manner:

- *Environmental barriers.* Having noise in the background or limited privacy, for instance, makes a truly empathic experience unlikely.
- *Time constraints.* The pharmacist (or the patient) may have limited time for the conversation; impatience is not conducive to communicating care.
- *Pharmacist-specific factors.* The pharmacist may feel uncomfortable or unprepared to engage with the patient's emotions. Another factor is the temptation to judge the patient's behavior. If the pharmacist is judgmental, it makes it harder to see the patient's perspective and gain his or her trust.
- *Patient-specific factors.* The patient must be interested in and ready to have a truly empathic exchange of thoughts and emotions with the pharmacist.
- *Lack of a relationship foundation.* Relationships take time to build. Without an existing relationship, the pharmacist may need to gather information about the patient to better understand his or her situation, as well as to establish trust and rapport.

EMPATHY AND BURNOUT

In *Professionalism, Work, and Clinical Responsibility in Pharmacy*, Tipton (2014) argues that because pharmacists, like other professional service providers, often have to regulate their own emotions in order to respond to their patients' emotional needs, problems such as burnout or compassion fatigue may occur. The author recommends that healthcare professionals strive to maintain a healthy balance between their own health and morale while responding to the needs of their patients. Similarly, a 2012 article by Zenasni, Boujut, Woerner, and Sultan presented three hypotheses regarding the possible relationships between provider empathy and burnout in a primary care setting. Empathy may create burnout, burnout may hamper empathy, or empathy may protect providers from experiencing burnout. The authors concluded that to achieve the third outcome, the ideal approach may be **clinical empathy**, which requires the provider's cognitive effort and ability to understand the patient's perspectives and experiences and to communicate that understanding and caring to the patient without being misplaced in the patient's pain and emotions. As a pharmacist, it is important to practice empathy when communicating with patients without jeopardizing your own emotional needs.

LEARN, PRACTICE, AND ASSESS
CASE STUDY EXERCISES

 LEARN: Example Patient Dialogues

Directions: Read the following case study. After completing Patient Dialogue One and Patient Dialogue Two, consider the differences between them and answer the questions provided.

PATIENT CASE

A 54-year-old Caucasian male presents for follow up to the local free health clinic where you are the clinical pharmacist. He was recently discharged from the hospital after a left big toe amputation resulting from uncontrolled diabetes and an infected ingrown toenail left untreated.

Social history: He has been unemployed for the past 3 years due to falling from a ladder while doing construction work and has been unsuccessful in obtaining disability compensation. He has no form of insurance and is grateful for the free health clinic's services. He takes care of his 72-year-old mother, who has Alzheimer's disease, and who was recently diagnosed with bone cancer and given 3 months to live. Many of his bills are at least 3 months past due, and he has not been able to pay the rent for his apartment for the past 4 months. His landlord has given him 3 weeks to move out or risk being evicted. He is severely depressed and stressed and does not care about his health. The one person in his life who cared about him, his mother, is getting worse every day and hardly remembers who he is. He just wants to lie around and eat junk food and has stopped checking his blood sugar. He can barely afford groceries, so he typically eats chips for breakfast, canned soup for lunch, and ramen noodles for dinner. He showers once a week.

PATIENT DIALOGUE ONE

Pharmacist: Hello, Mr. Martin. It is nice to see you again. Please have a seat here. We will start off by getting your vitals and a list of your medications.

Patient: (*Walks in looking down to the ground and speaks with a nonchalant demeanor.*) Hi (*still avoiding eye contact*).

Pharmacist: (*Takes blood pressure, pulse, and respiratory rate and blood glucose.*) Your blood pressure is a little high today and your blood sugar is really high. What is going on?

Patient: A lot is going on. I just don't care anymore about my health.

Pharmacist: Mr. Martin, if you don't care about your health, who else will? You have to start making better choices. Have you been checking your blood sugar?

Patient: No.

Pharmacist: Why not? The doctor is not going to be happy with your blood pressure *and* your blood sugar. Let's go through your medications. (*The patient hands the pharmacist a list of his medications and she records them in his chart.*) Are there any problems you want me to make the doctor aware of in your chart? You said there is a lot going on.

Patient: No, I really don't want to talk about it (*tears roll down his face*). I just want to be seen by the doctor. I have another appointment I need to get to after this one.

Pharmacist: (*Hands patient a tissue.*) I'm sorry you are upset. I will get you over to see the doctor. I hope things get better for you. See you next time. (*The patient walks out the door.*)

PATIENT DIALOGUE TWO

Pharmacist: Hello, Mr. Martin. It is nice to see you again. Please have a seat here. We will start off by getting your vitals and a list of your medications.

Patient: (*Walks in looking down to the ground and speaks with a nonchalant demeanor.*) Hi (*still avoiding eye contact*).

Pharmacist: (*Picks up the blood pressure cuff, getting ready to take his blood pressure.*) Mr. Martin, you don't seem like yourself today. What is bothering you? (*Leans in to the patient to actively listen.*)

Patient: A lot is going on. I just don't care anymore about my health.

Pharmacist: (*Puts down the blood pressure cuff.*) This can wait, let's talk about what is bothering you.

Patient: (*Makes eye contact with the pharmacist and his eyes start to tear up.*) You have no idea how stressed I am right now! My mom has bone cancer and the doctors say she only has 3 months to live. (*He gets upset and starts to cry harder.*)

Pharmacist: (*Hands the patient some tissue and leans in toward the patient.*) Mr. Martin, I am so sorry about your mom. I understand how upsetting this is for you. I am here to listen if you want to talk more about this.

Patient: My mother is really my only family at this point, and she has lived with me for the last 15 years; the thought of possibly losing her so quickly is just too much to bear. Seeing her in so much pain just makes me want to forget about my own health and be there for her.

Pharmacist: I remember when my grandmother was told she had breast cancer and it started to spread to other parts of her body. Our family was very upset about this news, but we knew that we had to be strong for her and help her get through it. So I wonder, Mr. Martin, if at this point taking care of your own health is the best thing you could do for your mother and yourself?

Patient: You are right. She is depending on me.

Pharmacist: Yes, she is depending on you, even though she may not be able to say it, and because of that we have to work on getting your diabetes under control.

(The patient starts to feel better, and they continue discussing his other social concerns regarding paying his rent and possibly getting evicted. The pharmacist offers a list of resources to assist him with food, paying bills, and temporary housing. The pharmacist obtains vital signs, medication and medical history, and provides patient education.)

Patient: I really appreciate you taking the time to listen and help me to deal with everything that is going on. You have no idea how much better I feel and how much this means to me.

Pharmacist: I am glad to help. Take care and I will see you in a month.

Discussion Questions for the **LEARN** Exercise

1. This text discusses empathy as a three-phase process. In what ways are the three phases illustrated in the patient dialogues? Do you see the different phases in Dialogue One? What about Dialogue Two?
2. Which verbal and nonverbal cues did Mr. Martin give that indicated his emotional distress? Do you think the pharmacist in Dialogue One noticed those cues? What about Dialogue Two?
3. Consider what the pharmacist did in Dialogue One. She did ask what was going on and said she was sorry the patient was upset. She also gave him a tissue when he started crying. Was that sufficient to communicate empathy to Mr. Martin? Why or why not?
4. In Dialogue Two, how did the pharmacist communicate to Mr. Martin that she was with him and would like to listen to what he had to say?
5. Why did the pharmacist in Dialogue Two tell Mr. Martin about her grandmother? In what ways might that have helped the pharmacist achieve her goal in the dialogue?

LEARN, PRACTICE, AND ASSESS   ● ▲ ■
CASE STUDY EXERCISES

▲ PRACTICE: Build Your Own Dialogue

Directions: Now it is time to *practice* what you have learned about the topic of this chapter. Reflecting on concepts from this chapter and the patient dialogues in the LEARN exercise, develop your own pharmacist–patient dialogue using the following patient information and guidance questions.

PATIENT CASE

A 37-year-old African-American woman with uncontrolled hypertension and uncontrolled type 2 diabetes presents to the free health clinic where you are the clinical pharmacist for a follow-up visit with her primary care physician. As the pharmacist, you complete the intake interview in which you obtain a complete medication history, vitals, and patient medical complaints. During the interview, she discusses a new medical issue that she is experiencing with her gums. She states that her gums are swollen, red, and tender. She has not seen a dentist in almost 10 years and she can only eat soft foods. She begins to cry as she discusses her husband leaving her recently, how she has become depressed because of her health, and that she feels her husband left her for another woman who is much prettier and smaller than she.

As you plan your dialogue, keep in mind what you have learned about communicating empathy to patients. Use the following questions to help plan and assess your dialogue.

1. An important part of planning a dialogue is setting goals for the conversation. Given the patient's situation, what would you like to accomplish in this dialogue? Be sure to think about both short- and long-term goals. For instance, you may want to calm her and stop her crying, but a more important goal is to communicate that you are with her and would like to listen to what she has to say.
2. As your patient begins to cry, what might you do or say in response to her emotional state?
3. We learned about communicating empathy to a patient using verbal and nonverbal strategies. While comforting and counseling this patient, which nonverbal and verbal cues can you use?
4. According to Barrett-Lennard (1993), empathy as a communicative process consists of three phases. In the last phase, the recipient—the

patient in this case—feels understood and comforted as a result of what is communicated by the other person. How would you know if your effort to communicate with empathy has worked? Which signals might the patient give that could help you decide if your empathic communication has worked?

5. As you plan your dialogue, have you considered any possible barriers for communicating empathy? How might you address them in your conversation?

YOUR DIALOGUE HERE

LEARN, PRACTICE, AND ASSESS
CASE STUDY EXERCISES

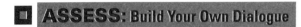

Directions: Now it is time to *assess* what you have learned about the topic of this chapter. In this exercise, no guidance questions are provided. Reflect on what you have learned from the LEARN and PRACTICE exercises, and develop your own pharmacist–patient dialogue using the following patient information.

PATIENT CASE

A 42-year-old Caucasian woman with uncontrolled hypertension, depression, and history of type 2 diabetes and two previous transient ischemic attacks presents to the ambulatory care clinic concerned about her blood pressure. She requests to be seen by the clinical pharmacist before she sees the physician because she enjoys talking with the pharmacist. As the pharmacist, you complete the intake interview in which you obtain a complete medication history, vitals, and patient medical complaints. During the interview, the patient discusses her worsening depression, which has caused her to regress back to hoarding. She confesses with obvious embarrassment that she only takes a bath once weekly and she has dishes piled up in her sink from last week. Her blood pressure in the clinic today is 156/98 (the patient's blood pressure goal is less than 140/80). She feels like she just wants to give up on everything.

YOUR DIALOGUE HERE

DISCUSSION QUESTIONS

1. Empathy was first studied in the field of psychotherapy and has since been studied and taught in the fields of medicine, nursing, and others. Consider the field of pharmacy. Compared to other healthcare providers, what unique challenges do pharmacists face when displaying empathy while interacting with patients?
2. Consider the environment where you practice or would like to practice. Which barriers, if any, exist that limit empathic communication? What would you do to remove these barriers?
3. Which personality traits and/or personal characteristics do you possess that may enhance or inhibit your ability to effectively display empathy?
4. This text discusses three possible relationships between empathy and provider fatigue. Have you observed examples of each relationship? How might one develop and display clinical empathy?

REFERENCES

Barrett-Lennard, G. T. (1993). The phases and focus of empathy. *British Journal of Medical Psychology, 66*(1), 3–14.

Hojat, M., Mangione, S., Gonnella, J. S., Nasca, T., Veloski, J. J., & Kane, G. (2001). Empathy in medical education and patient care [Letter to the editor]. *Academic Medicine, 76*(7), 669.

Lussier, M-T., & Richard, C. (2007). Feeling understood: Expression of empathy during medical consultations. *Canadian Family Physician, 53*(4), 640–641.

Mercer, S. W., & Reynolds, W. J. (2002). Empathy and quality of care. *British Journal of General Practice, 52*, 9–12.

Montague, E., Chen, P-Y., Xu, J., Chewning, B., & Barrett, B. (2013). Nonverbal interpersonal interactions in clinical encounters and patient perceptions of empathy. *Journal of Participatory Medicine, 5*. Retrieved from http://www.jopm.org/evidence/research/2013/08/14/nonverbal-interpersonal-interactions-in-clinical-encounters-and-patient-perceptions-of-empathy/

Nightingale, S. D., Yarnold, P. R., & Greenberg, M. S. (1991). Sympathy, empathy, and physician resource utilization. *Journal of General Internal Medicine, 6*(5), 420–423.

Tipton, D. (2014). *Professionalism, work, and clinical responsibility in pharmacy.* Burlington, MA: Jones & Bartlett Learning.

Zenasni, F., Boujut, E., Woerner, A., & Sultan, S. (2012). Burnout and empathy in primary care. *British Journal of General Practice, 62*(600), 346–347.

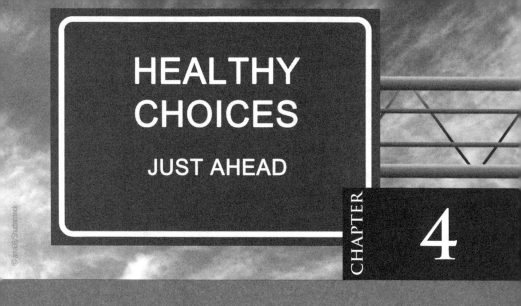

HEALTHY CHOICES

JUST AHEAD

CHAPTER 4

MOTIVATIONAL INTERVIEWING

LEARNING OBJECTIVES

At the end of this chapter, students should be able to:

▸ Define *motivational interviewing* (MI) in the context of healthcare practices.

▸ Understand the spirit of MI, the stages of change, the processes of MI, and the core communication skills associated with MI.

▸ Generate patient-centered communication strategies to elicit behavior change.

KEY TERMS

Action stage of change

Contemplation stage of change

Maintenance stage of change

Motivational interviewing (MI)

Precontemplation stage of change

Preparation stage of change

Chronic diseases are the leading cause of death and disability in the United States, resulting in 7 out of 10 deaths each year (U.S. Department of Health and

Table 4-1: Biomedical Approach Versus Motivational Interviewing Approach

Biomedical Approach to Care	Motivational Interviewing Approach to Care
Provider centered	Patient centered
Information giving	Information exchanged
Dictate behavior	Negotiate behavior
Provide motivation	Assess motivation
Resistance is seen as bad	Resistance is seen as useful information
Patient respect is expected	Patient respect is earned

Human Services, 2010). A patient's own behaviors and lifestyle are important to the prevention and management of chronic conditions (e.g., diabetes, heart disease) and determine his or her future health and quality of life (Rollnick, Miller, & Butler, 2008). Patient ambivalence about their own health and changes needed, such as behavioral change or treatment, is a key barrier for adherence. An example of patient ambivalence could be poor treatment adherence to antiretroviral therapy for HIV due to side effects, or a patient continuing to smoke cigarettes daily, despite being informed of the increased cardiovascular risk associated with smoking.

Motivational interviewing (MI) is a collaborative, person-centered communication style intended to elicit behavior change by helping patients explore and resolve ambivalence (Miller & Rollnick, 2013; Berger, 2005). Originally proposed in the context of addiction treatment, the model is now widely practiced across many healthcare disciplines. This chapter will review the spirit of MI, the stages of change, the process of MI, and the core communication skills associated with MI. It is important to understand that MI is an interpersonal style of communication and thus is not restricted to formal counseling settings. MI can be as brief as 15 minutes or a long as 1 hour and can be incorporated into all patient encounters by physicians, dentists, pharmacists, nurses, health educators, and therapists (Rollnick et al., 2008). One of the main principles of MI is that motivation to change is elicited from within the patient. It is important to understand that MI does not involve the manipulation or persuasion of a patient by the provider to elicit change. The provider–patient relationship should be more of a partnership than an expert–recipient role (Miller & Rollnick, 2013). **Table 4-1** highlights the general differences between the biomedical approach to providing care and the motivational interviewing approach.

THE SPIRIT OF MOTIVATIONAL INTERVIEWING

There are four key elements that experts have described as the spirit of MI: *partnership, acceptance, compassion,* and *evocation* (Miller & Rollnick, 2013; Berger, 2005). Communication is used to build a *collaborative partnership* among two experts: Pharmacists are the experts on medication therapy; patients are the experts on themselves. The chapter on the Pharmacist–Patient Relationship addresses this concept in more detail, highlighting the importance of honoring patient autonomy and self-direction and avoiding the urge to try to solve patients' problems for them. *Acceptance* can be conveyed through empathic listening and attempting to better understand the patient's perspective (see the chapter on Empathy and Patient Communication). To be *compassionate* is to value the well-being of the patient and to view life from his or her perspective (Miller & Rollnick, 2013. Finally, the pharmacist must be willing to suspend an authoritarian role and recognize that if change does occur, it needs to be the patient's choice. The MI provider's goal is to *evoke and strengthen change* that is already present from within the patient. Because pharmacy is a "helping profession," pharmacists may feel the desire to direct or tell patients how to improve their care. The righting reflex is the overwhelming desire to persuade a patient to "do the right thing" (Miller & Rollnick, 2002). Patients are often left feeling frustrated, defensive, uncomfortable, or powerless over their own care, and resistance to change will likely occur. When a patient is ambivalent about a treatment decision, it is not uncommon to hear two types of talk: change talk and sustain talk. Change talk is the patient's own statement indicating his or her reason for change (Miller & Rollnick, 2013). The use of MI is intended to increase change talk.

The following five questions related to smoking cessation are presented here to help you better understand the spirit of MI (Miller & Rollnick, 2009):

1. Why would you want to quit smoking?
2. How might you go about successfully quitting?
3. What are the three best reasons for you to quit?
4. How important is it for you to quit and why?
5. So what do you think you will do?

STAGES OF CHANGE

In the Transtheoretical Model of behavior change, five stages of change (see **Figure 4-1**) have been identified: precontemplation, contemplation, preparation, action, and maintenance (Prochaska & DiClemente, 1984). Readiness to change and progression through the stages of change often fluctuate over time. In the first stage, **precontemplation**, the patient is not ready to think about change or is unaware that there is a problem. **Contemplation** indicates that the patient is ready to think about change and may recognize his or her behavior as problematic. **Preparation** is the act of preparing for change, and **action** is actually implementing change. The last stage is **maintenance**, which is ensuring that the change in behavior becomes constant, with a focus

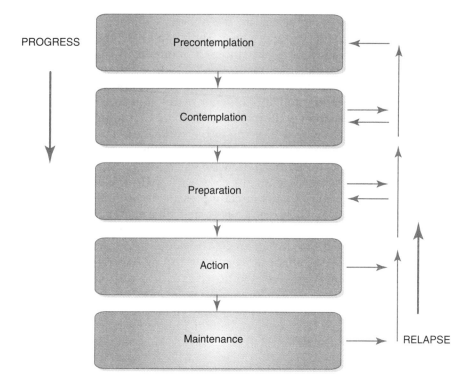

PROGRESS

Figure 4-1   Transtheoretical Model of Behavior Change

on preventing relapse into old behavior. In the context of addiction treatment, 80% of patients with substance use disorders are in a precontemplative or contemplative stage of change. During patient consultations, a pharmacist should gather information to ascertain which stage a patient may be in regarding the behavioral change and use the most appropriate communication strategies to motivate behavioral change.

FOUR (OVERLAPPING) PROCESSES OF MOTIVATIONAL INTERVIEWING

1. *Engaging.* Establishing a helpful and working relationship with the patient is the first step in MI. For some, this may occur immediately; for others it may take multiple encounters. Building a therapeutic relationship with the patient is necessary to promote successful change (Miller & Rollnick, 2013). During the engagement process, the pharmacist should attempt to better understand the patient's perspective and treatment concerns (express empathy).

2. *Focusing.* The pharmacist must maintain the focus of the conversation encompassing behavior change. This includes staying focused on the patient's self-described treatment plan goals. During this process, it is important to identify the patient's goals for change and to also consider whether they differ from your treatment goals (Miller & Rollnick, 2013).

3. *Evoking.* Eliciting the patient's own motivation for change is an important process in MI. Educating patients on what they are doing wrong and how to fix their problem will not evoke change. Instead, the pharmacist should help patients identify reasons that are meaningful for them. A method of evoking change is to use a scale ranging from 0 to 10 (Berger & Hudmon, 1997). "On a scale of zero to ten, with ten being the most important, how important would you say it is for you to quit smoking today?" Following up with a question about why the patient is a 5 and not a 2 or a 10 will likely evoke change talk. Another method of evoking change is to work with the patient to explore both the pros and cons of each option being considered (Hettema, Steele, & Miller, 2005).

4. *Planning.* The pharmacist should help the patient develop a plan for change. This is an ongoing process that should be revisited often. The pharmacist should determine what will help the patient move forward through active listening. The pharmacist should not develop or direct a plan for the patient without his or her input.

CORE COMMUNICATION SKILLS OF MOTIVATIONAL INTERVIEWING

There are five core communication skills that should be used throughout the process of MI (Miller & Rollnick, 2013).

1. *Ask open-ended questions* to build and strengthen the therapeutic relationship and gain knowledge surrounding ambivalence and change. Examples of open-ended questions include: "What brings you here today?" "Tell me about your daily routine." "How does your alcohol use affect your relationship with your husband?" Examples of closed-ended questions are: "Have you been checking your blood sugar regularly?" "Have you smoked cigarettes since our last session?" "Do you exercise routinely?"

2. *Affirm* and respect a patient's strengths. Emphasizing what a patient is doing wrong does not elicit behavior change. Examples of affirming statements include: "I appreciate your taking the time to meet with me today." "You really value your health." "You have made a lot of important progress."

3. *Reflect on* statements that a patient has made to ensure an understanding or clarify points of uncertainty. Reflective listening also allows patients to hear their statement again and think about its accuracy. You may repeat or slightly rephrase what the patient has said, or make inferences about what the patient has said, with the purpose of facilitating communication and moving the conversation forward (Miller & Rollnick, 2013), as can be seen in the following example:

Patient: "I can't quit smoking unless my boyfriend does too."

Pharmacist: "You can't imagine how you could not smoke with your boyfriend, and at the same time you're concerned about how it's affecting your health."

4. *Summarize* what the patient has said during your interaction to allow for reflection on his or her statements. This demonstrates that you are actively listening to the patient's concerns (Miller & Rollnick, 2013).

5. *Inform and advise* when a patient asks for it. Examples of information that a pharmacist could provide during a patient interaction include disease-state education, medication name, dosing, onset of action, and two or three common side effects. Following the spirit of MI, the patient is always free to disagree or to decide not to implement recommendations made by the pharmacist (Miller & Rollnick, 2009).

As you reflect on this discussion of the spirit of MI, its communication processes, and the various communication skills required to accomplish MI, keep in mind that MI is ultimately built on a true understanding of and respect for patient autonomy. For instance, in MI sessions, patient permission is requested before providing information. A simple approach for information exchange during a MI session is to follow the elicit-provide-elicit model (Miller & Rollnick, 2013). This involves first asking patients for permission to provide them with information, exploring their prior knowledge of the topic, and asking for their interpretation or understanding of the information you have provided. Methods such as this allow the pharmacist to earn the patient's trust and increase the chance of eliciting and maintaining change. This is why MI has been so well accepted and continues to be practiced as a key communication tool for motivating behavioral change.

LEARN, PRACTICE, AND ASSESS
CASE STUDY EXERCISES

 LEARN: Example Patient Dialogues

Directions: Read the following case study. After completing Patient Dialogue One and Patient Dialogue Two, consider the differences between them and answer the questions provided.

PATIENT CASE

Jamie Qualls is a 35-year-old married female who has been hospitalized for severe depression, anxiety, and suicidal thinking. She reported feeling depressed "off and on" since she was a teenager. She has tried antidepressant therapy in the past but does not like that she gained weight with use. Currently, she drinks one half to one full bottle of wine every night to "calm my nerves and sleep better." She also smokes one pack of cigarettes per day. She is unsure about taking another medication that may have side effects. On hospital discharge, the pharmacist is asked to discuss the newly prescribed sertraline (Zoloft) 50 mg daily with the patient in her room prior to her leaving the hospital.

PATIENT DIALOGUE ONE

Pharmacist: Hello, I am a pharmacist here at the hospital, and I would like to review your treatments with you before you are discharged.

Patient: Okay. I'm not a huge fan of taking meds, though.

Pharmacist: Understandable, but medications are really the best option for you right now for your depression. Why don't you want to take the Zoloft?

Patient: I didn't say that I didn't want to take it. I just don't want to gain weight.

Pharmacist: Weight gain is not a common side effect of this medication; nausea and a decrease in your sex drive are more common.

Patient: (*Rolling eyes.*) Oh, well, I don't know how I feel about that.

Pharmacist: I also see that you drink alcohol pretty regularly. You really shouldn't drink alcohol while taking this medication. It will make you feel more depressed and have a negative impact on your liver.

Patient: What? You're telling me I have to give up my wine, the one thing that helps my nerves, helps me stay calm, *and* helps me sleep? No way!

(The patient looks at the clock in a disinterested manner and walks toward the bathroom.)

Patient: I have to use the restroom. Can you let my nurse know that I am ready to leave now?

(The patient walks toward the bathroom and the pharmacist leaves the room frustrated with the patient.)

PATIENT DIALOGUE TWO

Pharmacist: Hello, I am a pharmacist here at the hospital, and I would like to review your treatments with you before you are discharged.

Patient: Okay. I'm not a huge fan of taking meds, though.

Pharmacist: I see that you have taken antidepressants in the past. Would you feel comfortable telling me about your previous experiences with antidepressants?

Patient: Sure. I took Remeron and I gained about 10 pounds! It is really important to me that I take a medication that doesn't cause that much weight gain.

Pharmacist: Your physical health is important to you. I am glad you brought this up. Would it be okay if I talked to you about the side effects of the new medication Zoloft compared to your previous medication Remeron?

Patient: I guess so (*with some hesitation*).

Pharmacist: Well, both are good treatment options for depression, but they work in different ways. Remeron is more likely to cause weight gain, but Zoloft is not known to cause significant weight gain. It can, however, cause some nausea initially and some people tell me that it negatively affects their sex drive. If this does occur, we have ways to treat this, so you may not have to stop your antidepressant. What do you think about what I have said so far?

Patient: I like that it doesn't cause a lot of weight gain, but I'm not a huge fan of it decreasing my sex drive. Thank you for taking the time to discuss the differences between the two.

Pharmacist: It's my pleasure. So, what do you think is the next step for you?

Patient: I think I would like to try taking the Zoloft. Can I ask you about taking it with alcohol? My doctor keeps pushing me to quit drinking and smoking, but I'm not sure I'm ready to do either.

Pharmacist: Of course, quitting both alcohol and cigarette use can be very challenging. Drinking alcohol along with an antidepressant can sometimes intensify the effects of the alcohol and can also decrease the antidepressant effect of the medication. Could you tell me more about how much you are drinking and smoking each day?

Patient: I drink about four glasses of wine every day and smoke about one pack per day. I am going to an alcohol treatment program when I leave the hospital, but I'm not so sure about quitting the whole smoking thing.

Pharmacist: Regarding your smoking, could you rate your readiness to quit smoking on a scale from one to ten, with ten indicating that you are ready to quit today?

Patient: I guess I would say that I am about a five.

Pharmacist: And why are you a five and not a three?

Patient: Well, I know I need to quit because it is bad for my health, but it calms me down so much when I am stressed. And I am afraid that I will gain weight if I stop cold turkey.

Pharmacist: Maintaining good health and weight is important to you and you're not sure where smoking falls with regard to your overall health. Would you be willing to explore alternative stress-reducing exercises other than smoking that could be helpful to you?

Discussion Questions for the **LEARN** Exercise

1. Which stage of change is the patient in, and did the pharmacist use appropriate MI skills given the stage she is in?
2. How does the pharmacist in Dialogue Two express empathy?
3. Compare the two dialogues. In what ways was change talk incorporated into the patient–pharmacist interaction in Dialogue Two?
4. How did the pharmacist in Dialogue Two use the key communication skills of MI as discussed in this text?

LEARN, PRACTICE, AND ASSESS
CASE STUDY EXERCISES

▲ PRACTICE: Build Your Own Dialogue

Directions: Now it is time to *practice* what you have learned about the topic of this chapter. Reflecting on concepts from this chapter and the patient dialogues in the LEARN exercise, develop your own pharmacist–patient dialogue using the following patient information and guidance questions.

PATIENT CASE

Gerry Rim is a 60-year-old husband and father of two adult children. He lives with his wife, and they stay fairly active spending time with their four grandchildren. He was diagnosed with diabetes and hypertension 10 years ago and takes metformin 1000 mg BID, glyburide 10 mg daily, and lisinopril 20 mg daily. His fasting blood glucose readings have steadily increased into the 200s, despite his current treatment. He has developed neuropathic pain in his feet that makes walking more difficult, and it is especially worse at night. His primary care physician initiated insulin therapy 1 month ago; however, Gerry has refused to begin the once-daily injection. The pharmacist is meeting with him at the Diabetes Treatment Center to discuss insulin injection techniques and address his questions and concerns about this new insulin treatment.

As you plan your dialogue, keep in mind what you have learned about MI. Use the following questions to help plan and assess your dialogue.

1. An important part of planning a dialogue is setting goals for the conversation. Given the patient's situation, what would you like to accomplish in this dialogue? Be sure to think about both short- and long-term goals. For instance, you may want to understand the patient's concerns with initiating insulin and motivate the patient to begin his insulin therapy as prescribed. At the same time, what would be a long-term goal for your conversation?
2. There are five stages of change. Assess which stage your patient identifies with and how you plan to move the patient to the next level of change.
3. There are five core communication skills that should be used throughout the process of MI. As you plan your dialogue, create an outline of those five skills and discuss how you plan to execute them.
4. Remember that motivational interviewing is a collaborative, person-centered communication style. Discuss ways you plan to display collaboration with the patient and how you will build a person-centered communication dialogue with the patient.

5. As you plan your dialogue, have you considered any possible barriers to behavioral change? How might you address them in your conversation?
6. Which verbal and nonverbal cues might the patient give you that MI is or is not working?

YOUR DIALOGUE HERE

LEARN, PRACTICE, AND ASSESS
CASE STUDY EXERCISES

☐ ASSESS: Build Your Own Dialogue

Directions: Now it is time to *assess* what you have learned about the topic of this chapter. In this exercise, no guidance questions are provided. Reflect on what you have learned from the LEARN and PRACTICE exercises, and develop your own pharmacist–patient dialogue using the following patient information.

PATIENT CASE

Theresa Tyson is a 51-year-old Caucasian female with severe alcohol dependence. She was recently diagnosed with alcoholic liver disease and has elevated liver function tests. She consumes approximately 15 drinks per day, including a mixture of beer and vodka throughout the day. She does not eat food because she states that she is never hungry due to obtaining her calories from alcoholic beverages. Her liver function is continuing to decline. She, along with her mother, are caretakers for her terminally ill sister and they live together. She presents to the clinic with yellowing of the eyes and skin and yellow discharge from her eyes. She also complains of right upper-quadrant abdominal pain that radiates to her back. The patient knows she needs to quit drinking but has not due to severe dependence, social stressors at home, and fear of alcohol withdrawal symptoms. The patient's psychiatrist is starting Librium 10 mg 1 tablet morning and afternoon and 2 tablets at night. The pharmacist is meeting with her to discuss her new medication and a plan for quitting drinking.

YOUR DIALOGUE HERE

DISCUSSION QUESTIONS

1. In the examples discussed in this chapter, MI is used to encourage patients who need to quit smoking and drinking. Discuss examples of other scenarios in which MI would be most effectively utilized by a pharmacist.
2. Consider the different processes discussed in this chapter such as engaging and evoking. What challenges or patient "pushback" might occur with each process? How would you respond if a patient pushes back in response to your engaging or evoking efforts, for instance?
3. Consider the five stages of the Transtheoretical Model discussed in this chapter. Why is it helpful to consider the specific stage your patient may be in when using MI for patient counseling?
4. Consider the typical working environment of a pharmacist in a community pharmacy or a hospital setting. Which barriers might make it challenging to use MI in patient encounters?

REFERENCES

Berger, B. A. (2005). *Communication skills for pharmacists: Building relationships, improving patient care* (2nd ed.). Washington, DC: American Pharmacists Association.

Berger, B. A., & Hudmon, K. S. (1997). Readiness for change: Implications for patient care, *Journal of the American Pharmaceutical Association, 37*(3), 321–329.

Hettema, J., Steele, J., & Miller, W. R. (2005). Motivational interviewing. *Annual Review of Clinical Psychology, 1*, 91–111.

Martino, S., Haeseler, F., Belitsky, R., Pantalon, M., & Fortin, A. H. (2007). Teaching brief motivational interviewing to year three medical students. *Medical Education, 41*(2), 160–167.

Miller, W. R., & Rollnick, S. (2002). Motivational interviewing: *Preparing people for change* (2nd ed.). New York, NY: Guilford Press.

Miller, W. R., & Rollnick, S. (2009). Ten things that motivational interviewing is not. *Behavioral and Cognitive Psychotherapy, 37*(2), 129–140.

Miller, W. R., & Rollnick, S. (2013). *Motivational interviewing: Helping people change* (3rd ed.). New York, NY: Guilford Press.

Prochaska, J. O., & DiClemente, C. C. (1984). *The transtheoretical approach: Crossing the traditional boundaries of therapy.* Malabar, FL: Kreiger.

Rollnick, S., Miller, W. R., & Bulter, C. C. (2008). *Motivational interviewing in health care: Helping patients change behavior.* New York, NY: Guilford Press.

U.S. Department of Health and Human Services. (2010). *Healthy People 2020.* Washington, DC: Author.

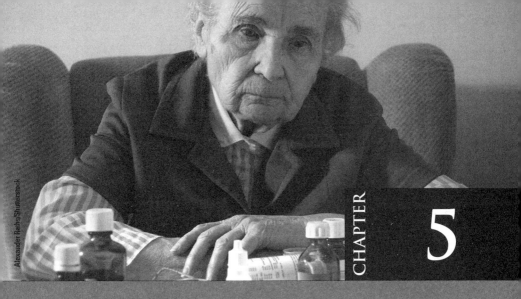

CHAPTER 5

MEDICATION ADHERENCE AND PATIENT COMMUNICATION

LEARNING OBJECTIVES

At the end of this chapter, students should be able to:

▸ Recognize poor medication adherence as a public health problem.

▸ Discuss the pharmacist's role and responsibilities in improving medication adherence.

▸ Apply the Health Belief Model to analyze the problem of poor adherence and generate solutions.

▸ Discuss general communication strategies to assess and improve patient adherence.

KEY TERMS

Adherence

Medication nonadherence

Former U.S. Surgeon General C. Everett Koop famously said, "Drugs don't work in patients who don't take them." Poor adherence to prescribed medication treatment is a costly public health problem with complex causes. A 2009 report of the Network for Excellence in Health Innovation concluded that poor patient medication adherence costs $290 billion annually in increased medical costs, in addition to poorer health, more frequent hospitalizations, and a higher risk of death. To fully understand the severity of this problem, consider the following statistics provided by the Centers for Disease Control and Prevention in 2013:

- Twenty percent to 30% of prescriptions are never filled.
- Of the billions of prescriptions dispensed in the United States annually, half are not taken as prescribed.
- Only half of Americans treated for hypertension adhere to their long-term therapy.
- Medication nonadherence is believed to cause 30% to 50% of treatment failures and 125,000 deaths annually.
- Improved self-management of chronic conditions results in a cost-to-savings ratio of 1:10.

ADHERENCE ISSUES: CONTRIBUTING FACTORS

Adherence is defined as the extent to which patients follow the instructions they are given for prescribed treatments. **Medication nonadherence** includes delaying prescription refills, failing to fill prescriptions, cutting dosages, and reducing or changing the frequency of administration. For decades, researchers and practitioners have tried to understand the causes of poor or nonadherence. Patients who are concerned with unpleasant side effects, confused about the medication, forgetful, have language barriers, or feel they no longer need the medicine are less likely to follow their medication regimen. Those with chronic conditions such as diabetes and high blood pressure also tend to have low adherence. What complicates this issue is that it is unlikely to find two patients with the exact same reasons for nonadherence.

A 2003 World Health Organization report on medication adherence argues that adherence is a multidimensional phenomenon shaped by five sets of factors. As shown in **Figure 5-1**, four of the five categories are factors that are not controlled by the patient, including *social/economic factors* (such as socioeconomic status, education level, and their living conditions), *condition-related factors* (such as severity of symptoms, comorbidities, and availability of effective treatments), *therapy-related factors* (complexity of the medical regimen, duration of treatment, immediacy of beneficial effects, and side effects), and *healthcare team and system-related factors* (such as insurance plan coverage, healthcare provider training, and the capacity of the system to educate and empower patients).

The category of *patient-related factors* is arguably the most important to pharmacists, as these factors are relatively easy to assess and possible to change through a pharmacist's effort. Examples of patient-related factors are knowledge, resources, attitudes, beliefs, motivation level, perceptions, and expectations. While pharmacists can benefit from understanding these four categories of contributing factors, there is little that individual pharmacists can do to help. However, with these patient-related factors, pharmacists can provide information to educate and empower patients, change these factors, and improve adherence.

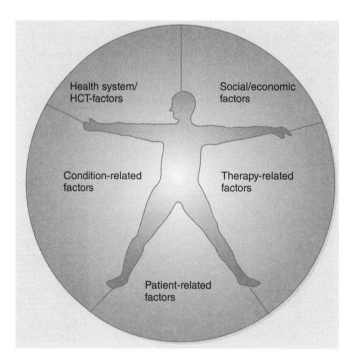

Figure 5-1   The Five Dimensions of Adherence

THE PHARMACIST'S ROLE IN PROMOTING ADHERENCE

Pharmacists have a unique responsibility and opportunity to discuss with their patients the importance of medication adherence and increasing adherence. From the patient's perspective, taking a pill as prescribed and following a medication regimen is a multistep effort, including (1) meeting with physicians and understanding medication needs; (2) receiving and understanding a treatment plan; (3) filling the prescription at a pharmacy; (4) taking the medication as prescribed; (5) managing the medication, which sometimes requires refills and follow-up consultation with healthcare providers; and (6) overall monitoring of one's medication use. A pharmacist's consultation is needed in many of these steps. In their communication with patients, pharmacists can identify potential barriers to adherence and use clear, supportive, and empowering communication to increase patient adherence.

THEORETICAL CONSIDERATIONS

The Health Belief Model offers a theoretical framework useful for understanding the underlying causes for low and nonadherence. A more complete review of this theory and its application to explaining health decision making is available in Glanz, Rimer, and Lewis (2002). Only when we have an educated understanding of why a problem exists can we then become part of the solution.

The Health Belief Model poses that an individual's health-related behavior, such as exercising or taking a medication, is influenced by a variety of factors (see **Figure 5-2**).

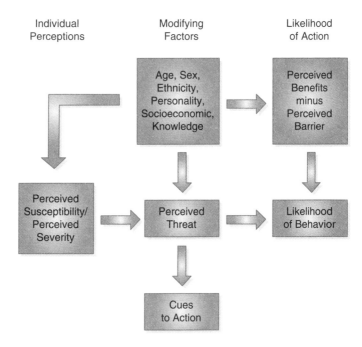

Figure 5-2 Health Belief Model

This model reminds us that a patient's likelihood of following a medication regimen is influenced by:

1. The extent to which a patient believes that he or she is likely to suffer from a negative health outcome unless something is done and that this negative health outcome is severe or life threatening.
2. The extent to which the patient believes that following the medication regimen will prevent the negative health condition or outcome (such as having a second heart attack).
3. The extent to which the patient feels that he or she can successfully follow the recommended medication regimen (i.e., barriers such as prohibitive cost may exist).

This model has been successful in predicting patient medication adherence. In one meta-analysis of 116 articles on medication adherence, patients' belief of the severity of the disease being treated or prevented significantly predicted patient adherence (DiMatteo, Haskard, & Williams, 2007).

The Health Belief Model suggests that during patient counseling, pharmacists should focus on the following tasks to encourage patient adherence:

1. Ensuring that patients understand their health condition, including the severity of the potential negative outcomes if the medication regimen is not followed.
2. Ensuring that patients understand what is prescribed, what the medication is for, and, if needed, offering an explanation of how the medication works to improve health.
3. Discussing any potential barriers (such as a complicated regimen and possible side effects) that may prevent patients from taking the medication on time.
4. Assessing the patient's overall confidence in taking the medication.
5. Offering medication devices such as calendars to help patients better manage their medication plan.

LEARN, PRACTICE, AND ASSESS
CASE STUDY EXERCISES

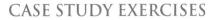
LEARN: Example Patient Dialogues

Directions: Read the following case study. After completing Patient Dialogue One and Patient Dialogue Two, consider the differences between them and answer the questions provided.

PATIENT CASE

Jim Adams is a 47-year-old Caucasian male who presents to his local pharmacy to pick up his wife's medications. His last self-blood pressure check at the pharmacy using an automatic cuff was 142/92.

- PMH: Hypertension x 5 years
- Medications: Lisinopril 20 mg 1 tablet po daily, OTC Tylenol 500 mg 1 tablet po prn arthritis pain

Jim's older brother recently had a heart attack and Jim is nervous that he may have a heart attack, but he does not know the possible causes. He thinks that his brother had a heart attack because he eats "bad." Jim forgets to take his blood pressure medication at least once a week and does not take the medication if his blood pressure is "normal," in the 140s/90s. Jim does not understand the importance of taking his blood pressure medication regularly.

PATIENT DIALOGUE ONE

Pharmacist: Hello, Mr. Adams. How are you doing today?

Patient: I'm doing all right. My brother had a heart attack last week so it has been a rough week. I just came in to pick up Judy's medicine for her.

Pharmacist: I'm sorry to hear that. Is your brother doing okay now?

Patient: Yeah, he's doing okay. He's back home now. Kind of scary, though, because he's only 55 and never been sick in his life.

Pharmacist: I see . . . I've got Judy's medication here; did you need anything for yourself today, Jim?

Patient: I don't think so, but you can check.

Pharmacist: Well, Jim, it looks like you haven't filled your lisinopril in the last two months. Would you like me to get it filled for you today?

Patient: No, I don't think so, because I think I still have some left.

Pharmacist: Oh, okay. If you have questions, be sure to give us a call.

Patient: Thank you.

PATIENT DIALOGUE TWO

Pharmacist: Hello, Mr. Adams. How are you doing today?

Patient: I'm doing all right. My brother had a heart attack last week so it has been a rough week. I just came in to pick up Judy's medicine for her.

Pharmacist: I'm sorry to hear that. Is your brother doing okay now?

Patient: Yeah, he's doing okay. He's back home now. Kind of scary, though, because he's only 55 and never been sick in his life.

Pharmacist: Wow, that is pretty scary. I've got Judy's medication here. Did you need anything for yourself today, Jim?

Patient: I don't think so, but you can check.

Pharmacist: Well, Jim, it looks like you haven't filled your lisinopril in the last 2 months. Did your doctor tell you to stop taking that medication?

Patient: No, he didn't, but I think I still have some left.

Pharmacist: Well, why don't I go ahead and get that ready for you, because you should be taking it daily.

Patient: That's okay, I really don't think I need to be taking it anyway, and I don't want to spend the money on it yet because I'm going to talk to him about stopping it.

Pharmacist: Do you know what you are taking that medication for?

Patient: I think it was because my blood pressure was a little high.

Pharmacist: That's right, Jim; it's for your high blood pressure. Have you been taking your medication every day?

Patient: Well, not exactly. I take it when I remember or when I notice my blood pressure is kind of high. I just don't think it's that serious to have to take it all of the time.

Pharmacist: I see. Did your doctor explain to you why it is important for you to take this medication?

Patient: Well, I mean he told me I should take it so my blood pressure goes down because he was afraid it was going to get too high and because of some kind of other heart problems.

Pharmacist: That is true; the medication is used to lower your blood pressure, but it is only effective if you take the medication every day. We want to lower your blood pressure by using this medication to prevent you from developing a more serious cardiac condition, including heart attack and stroke.

Patient: You mean having high blood pressure could cause me to have a heart attack like my brother?

Pharmacist: Yes, high blood pressure increases the risk for cardiovascular disease and can increase your risk for having a heart attack, stroke, or heart failure. The fact that your brother has had a heart attack at such a young age also puts you at risk for developing one of these conditions.

Patient: I didn't know that high blood pressure could cause a heart attack. I don't want to have to go through what my brother has gone through. Could you go ahead and get that medication ready for me?

Pharmacist: Sure, Jim, I can get that ready for you. Would you like to set up a time so we can talk about some other things you can do to decrease your risk of having a heart attack as well?

Patient: I think that might be a good idea. I had no idea how serious high blood pressure could be.

Discussion Questions for the **LEARN** Exercise

1. The Health Belief Model illustrates that a patient's likelihood to adhere to a medication regimen is influenced by several factors, such as perceived threat and perceived benefit. Use the theory to explain why the patient was not adhering to his blood pressure medication. Do you think the pharmacist in Dialogue Two addressed the right reasons? Please explain.

2. The pharmacist in Dialogue One missed an opportunity to educate this patient about his medication and as a result the patient left without realizing that his health is at great risk. Knowing the common risk factors for medication nonadherence, how do you plan to prevent making the same mistake?

3. The patient admitted that he stopped taking the medication when he felt that his blood pressure was improving. Many patients do the same thing, stopping their medications prematurely when symptoms start to go away. The pharmacist in Dialogue Two did not really address this issue. How would you explain to a patient the importance of taking a blood pressure medication or an antibiotic, even when no longer experiencing the symptoms?

4. The patient is in his late 40s. Patients of different age groups may face different issues related to medication adherence. If this patient was in his late 70s, should the pharmacist consider different factors and use different strategies to improve adherence? Please explain.

LEARN, PRACTICE, AND ASSESS
CASE STUDY EXERCISES

 PRACTICE: Build Your Own Dialogue

Directions: Now it is time to *practice* what you have learned about the topic of this chapter. Reflecting on concepts from this chapter and the patient dialogues in the LEARN exercise, develop your own pharmacist–patient dialogue using the following patient information and guidance questions.

PATIENT CASE
Ryan Stacks is a 49-year-old male with a recent diagnosis of type 2 diabetes. His HgA1C at diagnosis was 8.2%. He was recently prescribed Metformin 500 mg twice daily and was instructed to increase to 1000 mg twice daily after 2 weeks. He started taking the new medication 2 weeks ago but stopped taking the evening dose because he was waking up in the middle of the night with diarrhea. He noticed that he was feeling better even on just the once-daily dose of Metformin so he self-discontinued the evening dose and did not double the Metformin dose as instructed. The patient cancelled his follow-up appointment that was scheduled for today with the clinical pharmacist and physician. The clinical pharmacist follows up with the patient by phone to discuss the importance of monitoring his blood glucose readings and his medication adherence.

As you plan your dialogue, keep in mind what you have learned about medication adherence and patient communication. Use the following questions to help plan and assess your dialogue.

1. An important part of planning a dialogue is setting goals for the conversation. Given the patient's situation, what would you like to accomplish in this dialogue? Be sure to think about both short- and long-term goals. For instance, you may want to understand why he stopped taking the Metformin and determine whether he is aware of what his blood glucose should be. However, a more important goal may be to communicate to him that you want to help him get his blood glucose under control and would like to listen to what he has to say.

2. What potential barriers to adherence exist for this patient? Consider all possible factors and address a few in your dialogue.

3. Patient-related factors for nonadherence are most important for pharmacists to address. Identify which patient-related factors exist for the patient and how you can address these factors. What information can you provide the patient to educate and empower him and improve his adherence?

4. According to the Health Belief Model, on which five key tasks should pharmacists focus to encourage patient adherence? Be sure to incorporate

these five tasks into your patient dialogue. How would you assess the success of your effort? What signals might the patient give that could help you decide if your communication was successful?

YOUR DIALOGUE HERE

LEARN, PRACTICE, AND ASSESS
CASE STUDY EXERCISES

 ASSESS: Build Your Own Dialogue

Directions: Now it is time to *assess* **what you have learned about the topic of this chapter. In this exercise, no guidance questions are provided. Reflect on what you have learned from the LEARN and PRACTICE exercises, and develop your own pharmacist–patient dialogue using the following patient information.**

PATIENT CASE

Kelly Martin, a 34-year-old Caucasian female, presents to the pharmacy to pick up a prescription refill for her Advair Diskus 250/50. The pharmacist notices that she is almost a month late with the refill and inquires about how she is using the inhaler. The patient states that she uses it when she is short of breath, usually once every day. Also, she was recently laid off from her job and tries to use the medication as infrequently as possible because it is expensive.

YOUR DIALOGUE HERE

DISCUSSION QUESTIONS

1. The World Health Organization (2003) report states that medication nonadherence is a multidimensional problem influenced by five categories of factors. As discussed in this text, four of the five categories are beyond the control of patients. Knowing this, what do you think pharmacists can do to help a patient who faces these factors?
2. This chapter ends with a list of tasks on which pharmacists can focus. Discuss with your class and add to the list any tasks that you think are missing.
3. Many patients use the Internet to search for health-related information. While a wealth of information could potentially increase health literacy for some, misinformation is a big problem. What medication adherence problems might this create for pharmacists as they communicate with patients?
4. Which protocols or tools are you aware of that pharmacies have in place to address the issue of medication nonadherence?
5. If you were to help a community pharmacy develop a new protocol to address medication nonadherence, which key elements should be included in the protocol?

REFERENCES

Centers for Disease Control and Prevention. (2013, March 27). *Medication adherence.* Retrieved from http://www.cdc.gov/primarycare/materials/medication/docs/medication-adherence-01ccd.pdf

DiMatteo, M. R., Haskard, K. B., & Williams, S. L. (2007). Health beliefs, disease severity, and patient adherence: A meta-analysis. Medical Care, 45(6), 521–528.

Glanz, K., Rimer, B. K., & Lewis, F. M. (Eds.). (2002). Health behavior and health education: Theory, research, and practice. San Francisco, CA: Jossey-Bass.

Network For Excellence in Health Innovation. (2009). *Improving patient medication adherence: A $290 billion opportunity.* Retrieved from http://www.nehi.net/bendthecurve/sup/documents/Medication_Adherence_Brief.pdf

World Health Organization. (2003). *Adherence to long-term therapies: Evidence for action.* Retrieved from http://whqlibdoc.who.int/publications/2003/9241545992.pdf

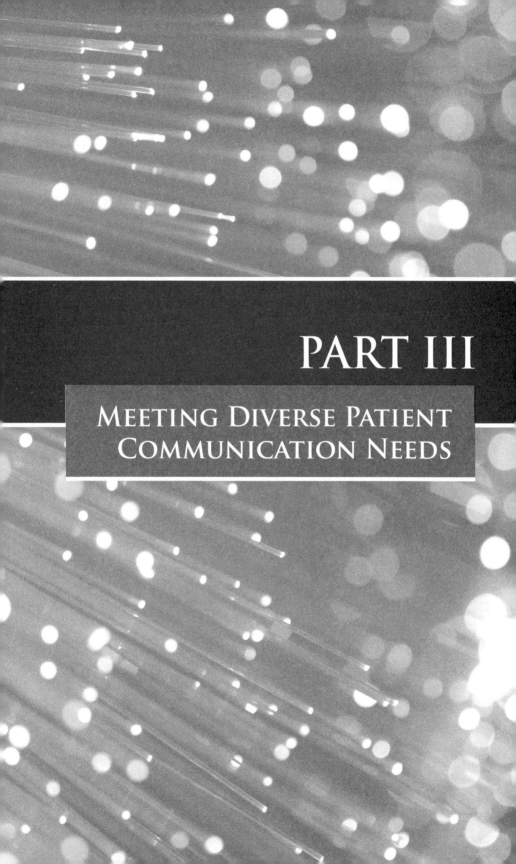

PART III

MEETING DIVERSE PATIENT COMMUNICATION NEEDS

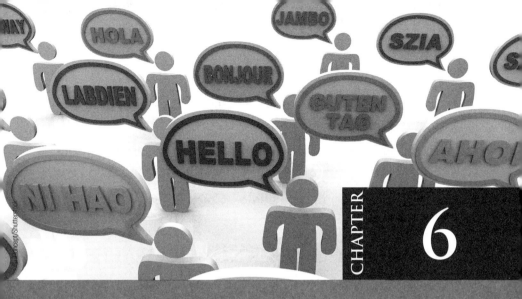

CHAPTER 6

CULTURAL COMPETENCY AND PATIENT COMMUNICATION

LEARNING OBJECTIVES

At the end of this chapter, students should be able to:

▸ Recognize cultural competency as an essential skill for pharmacy professionals.

▸ Apply the continuum of cultural competence in assessing one's own cultural competency level and setting goals.

▸ Apply the LEARN Model to generate communication strategies when communicating with diverse patients.

KEY TERMS

Cultural blindness

Cultural competence

Cultural destructiveness

Cultural incapacity

Cultural pre-competence

Cultural proficiency

Culture

At one point in your pharmacy training, you may have been asked the question, "Is it more important to know what sort of disease a patient has, or what sort of patient has the disease?" As Sir William Osler, a pioneer Canadian physician and one of the founding professors of John Hopkins Hospital, shrewdly stated, the latter is more important for a healthcare professional. It may also be arguably more difficult, especially when considering our diverse society and the multitude of factors that influence a patient's healthcare experience.

CULTURAL COMPETENCY IN HEALTH CARE AND PHARMACY

Cultural competency is an important and relevant topic for healthcare providers. Due to increasing diversity and population projections, pharmacists and other healthcare professionals must be prepared to provide individualized and culturally competent care to patients. By the year 2050, half of the U.S. population will be made up of minorities (Passel & Cohn, 2008). Treating all patients the same is not ideal; instead, patient care should be individualized. A patient's **culture** is his or her body of learned beliefs, traditions, and guides for behaving that are shared among members of a particular group. Culture involves all aspects of life, including values, beliefs, customs, communication styles, behaviors, practices, worldviews, clothing, art, and food preferences. Healthcare providers who are ignorant of their patients' cultural backgrounds will not achieve effective patient communication. A healthcare provider's bias against a patient because of cultural differences in values or beliefs can create a communication barrier and therefore deter the development of a meaningful patient–provider relationship. Patients who are not comfortable with their provider are less likely to share health information vital to properly assessing and treating conditions.

In 2000, the Office of Minority Health published the first National Standards for Culturally and Linguistically Appropriate Services in Health and Health Care (National CLAS Standards), which provided a framework for all healthcare organizations to best serve the nation's increasingly diverse communities; the standards were revised in 2010 (Office of Minority Health, n.d.). Four of the 15 standards focus on communication and language assistance. One standard states that healthcare organizations are to offer language assistance to individuals who have limited English proficiency and/or other communication needs at no cost to the patients. Pharmacies have many tools to choose from when serving their non-English-speaking clients, through written translation, verbal interpretation, or a combination of both. A 2011 study by Feichtl, Clauson, Alkhateeb, Jamass, and Polen surveyed 1,000 community pharmacies (both independent and chain pharmacies) and concluded that they are not consistently or optimally using language-access services. About 41% said they never used translation in their pharmacy, and 40% never used interpretation. Fear of potential inaccuracies and lack of time were cited as the primary reasons.

Between 2007 and 2013, the American College of Clinical Pharmacy (ACCP) published a five-part white paper series on cultural competency in health care and the implications for pharmacy. The papers synthesized the scholarship and provided a thorough review for best practices and implications for pharmacy education and policy related to cultural competency (ACCP, n.d.).

CONTINUUM OF CULTURAL COMPETENCE IN HEALTH CARE

The National CLAS Standards and the ACCP white papers mostly provide a blueprint for healthcare organizations, including pharmacies, to implement culturally and linguistically appropriate services. Let us consider what we as individuals can do to become culturally competent. The first step is to examine ourselves and consider what our strengths and limitations are when it comes to interacting with different cultural groups. The cultural competence continuum, presented in **Figure 6-1**, consists of six levels and is a useful tool for healthcare professionals when determining their cultural competence status and setting goals for professional development (Cross, Bazron, Dennis, & Isaacs, 1989). Discussion and application of this continuum can be found in many academic sources, including Campinha-Bacote (2007).

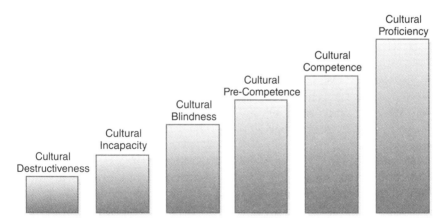

Figure 6-1   Continuum of Cultural Competence in Health Care

1. **Cultural destructiveness:** A lack of understanding of diverse cultures and an unwillingness to understand other cultures.
2. **Cultural incapacity:** A lack of capacity to respond effectively to culturally and linguistically diverse groups.

3. **Cultural blindness**: All people are viewed the same without taking into consideration their cultural differences.
4. **Cultural pre-competence**: A very preliminary stage where strengths and areas of growth of cultural competence are known, but progress has not yet been made to move forward.
5. **Cultural competence**: Confirming that the needs of diverse patients and customers are met, valuing diversity, and taking concrete steps to ensure efficacy in serving minority populations
6. **Cultural proficiency**: The highest level—active pursuit of resource development without hesitation.

Dr. Josepha Campinha-Bacote, a well-known scholar and consultant in the field of cultural competency in health care who proposed this continuum model, reminded practitioners to focus on the *process of becoming* more and more culturally competent, rather than approaching it as a *state of being*. In other words, being culturally competent with our patients on a daily basis is a continuous journey, mainly because our patient demographics are everchanging. We should not expect to finally *arrive at* cultural competency one day. Finishing a course or training, or even receiving a certification related to cultural competency, does not make us culturally competent practitioners; the key is to translate these principles into actual patient care behaviors, specifically with regard to how we communicate with patients from diverse backgrounds.

THE LEARN MODEL OF CULTURALLY COMPETENT COMMUNICATION

Several models have been proposed in medicine, nursing, counseling, and other related professions to serve as a framework for communicating with diverse patients in a culturally sensitive manner. Implementing the LEARN Model the next time you interview or counsel a patient may prove helpful, especially when cultural barriers may be causing some communication challenges.

The LEARN model, developed by Berlin and Fowkes (1983), provides a useful communication framework that pharmacists can implement in direct patient encounters (see **Figure 6-2**). The five steps of this model include:

1. *Listen.* In this step, you listen with empathy and focus on understanding the patient's perception of the health situation. Questions to ask may include, "What do you feel caused the health problems you are having?" "What do you feel might help you address the problems?" The pharmacist may focus on understanding what the patient has been doing to alleviate or improve the symptoms and why.

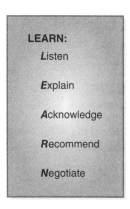

LEARN:
Listen

Explain

Acknowledge

Recommend

Negotiate

Figure 6-2   The LEARN Model

2. *Explain*. In this step, the practitioner explains the illness, diagnosis, and recommended treatment plan to the patient. The pharmacist may focus on explaining in clear, simple ways which medications are prescribed, how they are supposed to work, and how the patient is supposed to take them.

3. *Acknowledge*. In this step, the practitioner acknowledges the differences, if any, between the patient's interpretation of the situation and the medical professional's. If a patient expresses concerns about a prescription or decides not to fill, it is likely because he or she did not fully understand the diagnosis or is not convinced that the medication will work or is necessary. In this case, the pharmacist must understand these differences and work with the patient to identify areas of similarities (such as the shared goal of improving health) and explore mutually satisfying solutions.

4. *Recommend*. With the information collected in the first three steps, the practitioner makes a recommendation that fits the patient's unique circumstances or beliefs. For pharmacists, this may mean suggesting an alternative medication if the one originally prescribed by the physician is not acceptable to the patient due to culturally specific reasons.

5. *Negotiate*. This step focuses on negotiating with the patient a plan of action that is feasible for the patient and removes any cultural barriers that may be prohibitive. For pharmacists, this may include discussing specific things that may make a medication regimen difficult for the patient to follow, as well as understanding unique cultural beliefs, values, or practices that affect the patient's ability to follow the treatment plan.

LEARN, PRACTICE, AND ASSESS
CASE STUDY EXERCISES

 LEARN: Example Patient Dialogues

Directions: Read the following case study. After completing Patient Dialogue One and Patient Dialogue Two, consider the differences between them and answer the questions provided.

PATIENT CASE

Ramona Williams, a 57-year-old African-American female, presented to the emergency room complaining of chest pains and high blood pressure (180/110) and was hospitalized. She was recently laid off from her job, and when her insurance was no longer active, she could not afford her medications. She does not like going to the doctor and has limited trust of healthcare providers due to her father being involved in the Tuskegee Syphilis Study about 50 years ago. In addition, she was diagnosed with schizophrenia 10 years ago because she told her doctor she heard the voice of God.

- PMH: Hypertension
  - Schizophrenia?
- Current medications: No meds x 1 month

During the second day of her hospitalization, Ms. Williams was praying and meditating when the hospital pharmacist came to speak with her about her medications. She asks if the pharmacist can come back later because she is waiting to hear the voice of God regarding her illness. She states that God is a healer and can heal her body from this high blood pressure. The pharmacist returns 20 minutes later.

PATIENT DIALOGUE ONE

Pharmacist: Hello, Ms. Williams. I am Alex, the clinical pharmacist. I would like to talk to you about your medications. Is this a good time?

Patient: (*Smiling and seems happier than previously.*) Sure, please come in. I was praying when you came in earlier.

Pharmacist: So, your blood pressure has come down quite a bit from where it was when you came into the hospital. Dr. Johnson prescribed two medications for your high blood pressure and one medication for your cholesterol. I see here that you will be discharged from the hospital today. Before you leave, I'd like to talk to you about these medications, how they work, how to take them, possible side effects, and so on and so forth (*flipping the pages of materials as she talks*).

Patient: Well (*pause*), actually, as I was telling you earlier, I am not sure if I will be needing all of these pills. I feel much better now and very much at peace and— (*interrupted by the pharmacist*).

Pharmacist: But Ms. Williams, the symptoms you had yesterday, the chest pains and the 180/100 blood pressure, could have resulted in something much worse, like a heart attack or stroke. You need these medications to prevent damage to some of the important organs in your body, such as your heart, eyes, brain, and kidneys. The blood pressure medications work by decreasing the amount of water and salt your body holds onto, causing your blood vessels to open and letting the blood freely flow through them, and also preventing the heart from working so hard. You will take all three medications once daily. You can take them first thing in the morning with your breakfast.

Patient: (*Remaining quiet as the pharmacist goes over the medications; she is visibly uninterested in the information.*)

Pharmacist: (*Finally looks up at the patient from her list of information to cover.*) So we've discussed the three medications you will be taking and how to take them. Do you have any questions about what we went over, Ms. Williams?

Patient: No, I don't think so. I understand what you just said (*thinking to herself: "I am not sure if you understood what I was saying."*).

Pharmacist: Oh, okay. If you have questions, be sure to give us a call.

Patient: Thank you.

PATIENT DIALOGUE TWO

Pharmacist: Hello, Ms. Williams. I am Alex, the clinical pharmacist. I would like to talk to you about your medications. Sorry for the interruption earlier. Is this a good time?

Patient: (*Smiling and seems happier than previously.*) Sure, please come in. I was praying when you came in earlier.

Pharmacist: Sure. You mentioned that you were praying and waiting to hear the voice of God. I was wondering if you've had a chance to speak with our hospital chaplain? Some of my other Christian patients seem to have had a positive experience talking with him.

Patient: No, but that's a great suggestion. Thank you.

Pharmacist: Ms. Williams, I am really glad that your blood pressure is much lower than it was before. The symptoms you had yesterday, the chest pains and the 180/100 blood pressure, could have resulted in something much worse, like a heart attack or stroke. That's why we'd like to start on a few medications. Before I talk to you about these medications, can you tell me what *you* have been doing for your blood pressure?

Patient: (*Her face lights up and she seems pleasantly surprised.*) Wow, I have never had a doctor ask me that; usually, they just cut straight to the chase. Well, I have been praying and I know that God is a healer. He will heal my body. And I don't mean to be disrespectful, but I really don't feel like I need the medications. I am going to be okay (*very uplifted and at peace*).

Pharmacist: You seem so much happier when you talk about your spirituality and I think that's a wonderful thing. I can see that you feel much better today and I am happy for you. I would still like you to see our chaplain because what you said reminded me of a conversation that he had with another Christian patient when I was in the room. I don't remember everything he said but I do remember him saying that God can heal you in many ways, including prayers, medications, and even surgeries (*pausing for the patient's reaction*).

Patient: (*Nodding.*) That makes sense. I haven't thought about it, but I have heard that before.

Pharmacist: I don't know everything about Christianity, but hopefully you'll get a chance to talk to the chaplain before you leave today. I can ask the nurse to schedule a meeting for you if you'd like. But in the meantime, would it be okay if we take some time to talk about the medications the doctor prescribed for you? I'd like to make sure that you understand why we think they are important and how to take them if you *do* decide you want to. And I would highly recommend that you do because you need them to prevent damage to some of the important organs in your body, such as your heart, eyes, brain, and kidneys.

Patient: (*Seems more interested.*) Sure, please go ahead.

(The pharmacist explains the medications, including instructions and side effects, to the patient. She maintains constant eye contact with the patient to ensure understanding and pauses periodically to see if the patient has questions.)

Pharmacist: (*Looks up at the patient from her list of information to cover.*) We've discussed the three medications you will be taking and how to take them. At this point, do you have any questions about what we went over, Ms. Williams?

Patient: No, not really. I appreciate your taking the time to understand what's important to me today. I just want to say that I do know that high blood pressure is a serious problem, and I do want to get better. I love God but I am not ready to meet Him in Heaven just yet (*the pharmacist and patient laugh*). I want to do what's right for me without compromising my beliefs.

Pharmacist: Thank you for giving me the opportunity to talk with you. I really appreciate your honesty and openness. I'll go ahead and ask your nurse to call the chaplain. If you have questions about these medications, be sure to give me a call.

Patient: Thank you.

Discussion Questions for the **LEARN** Exercise

1. As we discussed in this chapter, when serving diverse patients, it is particularly important to listen to the patient and understand any beliefs and values that might be relevant to his or her healthcare needs. Which verbal and nonverbal strategies did the pharmacist in Dialogue Two use to persuade the patient to open up and share her beliefs and thoughts?
2. Use the LEARN Model to analyze the patient dialogues. Did the pharmacist in Dialogue Two go through all five steps?
3. Consider the pharmacist in Dialogue One. Which level of the cultural competency continuum do you think her communication represents? What about the pharmacist in Dialogue Two? What do you think are the most significant differences between the two dialogues?
4. The pharmacist in Dialogue Two uses the hospital chaplain as a resource to communicate with the patient regarding her spirituality. Another resource could be a certified health interpreter to assist a patient with limited English. What other resources in your organization or your community might you be able to call on to assist culturally diverse patients?

LEARN, PRACTICE, AND ASSESS
CASE STUDY EXERCISES

 PRACTICE: Build Your Own Dialogue

Directions: Now it is time to *practice* what you have learned about the topic of this chapter. Reflecting on concepts from this chapter and the patient dialogues in the LEARN exercise, develop your own pharmacist–patient dialogue using the following patient information and guidance questions.

PATIENT CASE

A family of three (father, mother, and 3-year-old child) are traveling to Florida for vacation and get into an automobile accident. All three family members are rushed to the local hospital for care. The mother and father are in stable condition but the child is in critical condition and has lost a significant amount of blood. The child requires a blood transfusion, and the doctor speaks with the parents about this medical need and asks for their signed consent. The parents state that this goes against their beliefs. Because the family is part of the Jehovah's Witness community, they would like the hospital to provide an alternative to the blood transfusion. The physician consults with the clinical inpatient pharmacist and the pharmacist is asked to speak with the family as soon as possible.

As you plan your dialogue, keep in mind what you have learned about culturally competent communication with patients. Use the following questions to help plan and assess your dialogue.

1. An important part of planning a dialogue is setting goals for the conversation. Given the patient's and family's situation, what would you like to accomplish in this dialogue? Be sure to think about both short- and long-term goals. For instance, you may want to understand the family's health beliefs and which blood products they are willing to accept for the child, but a more important goal may be to communicate to the family that you want to help their child get better while complying with their religious beliefs and would like to listen to what they have to say.
2. The first step in becoming culturally competent is examining yourself. What are your strengths and limitations when interacting with a Jehovah's Witness patient (assuming that you are not one)?
3. Using the LEARN Model, devise an outline of how you plan to incorporate the model into your dialogue (Listen, Explain, Acknowledge, Recommend, and Negotiate). Be sure to include the questions you plan to ask the patient's family.
4. What other resources can you consult in addition to the family to determine a recommendation for treatment? The family's religious leader may be contacted and could assist the family and pharmacist in

devising a treatment plan. How might the family feel about your plan if you as the pharmacist offer to include their religious leader in the discussion?

YOUR DIALOGUE HERE

LEARN, PRACTICE, AND ASSESS
CASE STUDY EXERCISES

 ASSESS: Build Your Own Dialogue

Directions: Now it is time to *assess* what you have learned about the topic of this chapter. In this exercise, no guidance questions are provided. Reflect on what you have learned from the LEARN and PRACTICE exercises, and develop your own pharmacist–patient dialogue using the following patient information.

PATIENT CASE

Jina Shim, 30 years old, has been hospitalized for a pregnancy-related complication. She is 4 months pregnant with her second child. The family practices Zen Buddhism, and Ms. Shim is strictly vegetarian. She does not eat the hospital food. As many Asian families do, Shim's family members bring her home-cooked food during her hospital stay. The first morning after her hospitalization, Shim's nurse arrives with her breakfast and medications, including a prenatal vitamin. Shim expresses strong concerns about the prenatal vitamins prescribed by her OBGYN because they have a fishy smell. Ms. Shim asks why prenatal vitamins are even needed, as no women in her family or her husband's family have ever taken them during their pregnancies and all gave birth to perfectly healthy children. For her, consuming only plant-based foods and vitamins is key to ensuring her child's health in this life and in future life cycles as well.

YOUR DIALOGUE HERE

DISCUSSION QUESTIONS

1. We often hear healthcare providers say, "I do not see skin color when I work with a patient. A diabetes patient is a diabetes patient whether an Asian patient or a Caucasian patient has it." Discuss your feelings about this perspective. Do you agree? Why or why not?
2. Which level of the cultural competence continuum do you most relate to? Why? Based on your current level, discuss how you plan to move further along the continuum.
3. As the National CLAS Standards suggest, providing culturally competent services to diverse patient populations requires commitment at the individual level as well as the organizational level. Consider the type of healthcare organization you work at or plan to work at. Which organizational policies and resources are in place to address the culturally diverse needs of the community?
4. Consider the demographic changes occurring in the United States and in your community. How might the ethnic and cultural makeup of your patients change in the coming decades? What additional skills will be required of pharmacists to meet these needs?

REFERENCES

American College of Clinical Pharmacy. (n.d.). *ACCP papers*. Retrieved from https://www.accp.com/govt/positionPapers.aspx

Berlin E. A., & Fowkes, W. C., Jr. (1983). A teaching framework for cross-cultural health care: Application in family practice. *Western Journal of Medicine, 139*(6), 934–938.

Campinha-Bacote, J. (2007). *The process of cultural competence in the delivery of healthcare services: The journey continues* (5th ed.). Cincinnati, OH: Transcultural C.A.R.E. Associates.

Cross, T. L., Bazron, B. J., Dennis, K. W., & Isaacs, M. R. (1989). *Towards a culturally competent system of care: A monograph on effective services for minority children who are severely emotionally disturbed.* Washington, DC: CASSP Technical Assistance Center, Georgetown University Child Development Center.

Feichtl, M. M., Clauson, K. A., Alkhateeb, F. M., Jamass, D. S., & Polen, H. H. (2011). Community pharmacists' use of language-access services in the United States. *Journal of the American Pharmacists Association, 51*(3), 368–372.

Office of Minority Health, U.S. Department of Health and Human Services. (n.d.). *CLAS and the CLAS standards.* Retrieved from https://www.thinkculturalhealth.hhs.gov/content/clas.asp

Passel, J. S., & Cohn, D. (2008, February 11). U.S. population projections: 2005–2050. *Pew Research Center.* Retrieved from http://www.pewhispanic.org/2008/02/11/us-population-projections-2005–2050/

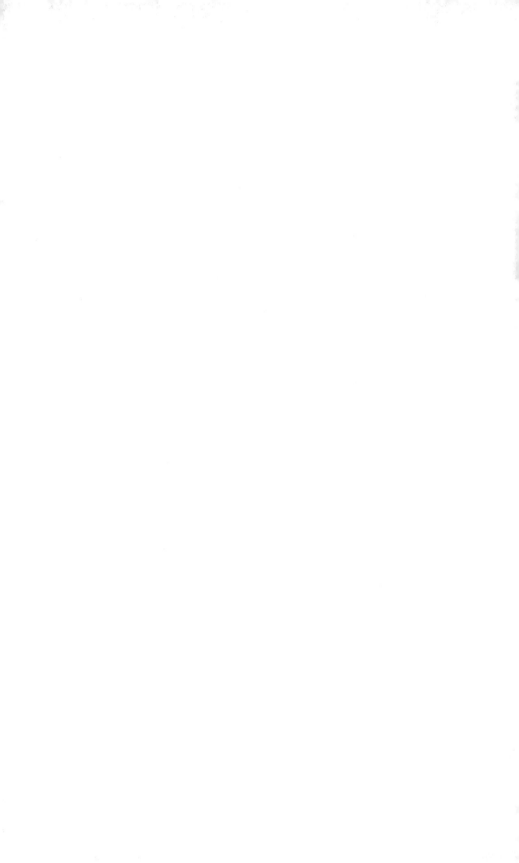

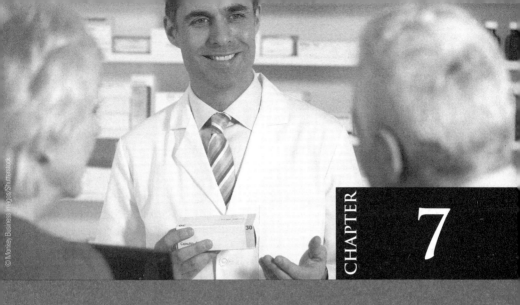

COMMUNICATING WITH LIMITED ENGLISH PROFICIENCY PATIENTS

LEARNING OBJECTIVES

At the end of this chapter, students should be able to:

▸ Describe language diversity patterns in the United States.

▸ Articulate the pharmacist's role and responsibilities for serving limited English proficiency (LEP) patients.

▸ Recognize federal- and state-level rules and regulations regarding language access for LEP patients.

▸ Discuss different communication access tools available for serving LEP patients.

▸ Discuss communication strategies to improve communication with LEP patients.

KEY TERMS

Limited English proficiency (LEP) individuals

America is a diverse nation, both culturally and linguistically. For instance, the Census Bureau (2013) codes 380 languages other than English to map the linguistic diversity within the nation. The proficiency of those who speak a language other than English may range from speaking English really well to speaking no English at all. To the surprise of many, English is not the official language for the United States; in fact, the country has no "official" language. Individuals who have limited English proficiency (LEP) face more challenges with daily activities, including communication with healthcare professionals. As a healthcare professional, you may find yourself interacting with patients and family members with varying levels of English proficiency. It is important to understand how to best serve their communication needs.

LANGUAGE NEEDS IN THE UNITED STATES

The federal interagency website www.lep.gov defines a **LEP individual** as someone who does not speak English as his or her primary language and has a limited ability to read, speak, write, or understand English. These individuals are entitled to language assistance with respect to healthcare services and encounters. U.S. Census Bureau (2013) data suggest that the percent of individuals in the United States who speak English less than "very well" grew from 8.1% in 2000 to 8.7% in 2011. To appreciate the importance of and challenges in communicating with LEP patients, consider the following facts based on 2013 census data:

- After English, Spanish is the language most commonly used at home (37.6 million), followed by Chinese (2.9 million).
- Other languages with at least 1 million users in the United States are Tagalog, Vietnamese, French, German, and Korean.
- English proficiency varies across language groups. Eighty percent or more of French and German speakers speak English "very well." In contrast, fewer than 50% of those who speak Korean, Chinese, or Vietnamese speak English "very well." The rate for Spanish speakers is 56%.
- Linguistic diversity exists in many areas around the world. For instance, the U.S. Census Bureau considers 8 Chinese language categories and 12 Indian language categories.

Language barriers affect the delivery of adequate care by causing poor exchange of information, misunderstanding of diagnosis and treatment information, poor shared decision making, and, most important, decreased adherence to medication and treatment plans (Agency for Healthcare Research and Quality, 2012).

LAWS AND REGULATIONS ON LANGUAGE SERVICES FOR LEP PATIENTS

The federal government is required to provide access to federal programs and federally assisted programs for LEP individuals (USA.gov, n.d.). Similarly, there are regulations and guidelines regarding language-access services that pharmacy professionals must provide for their LEP patients. The National Standards for Culturally and Linguistically Appropriate Services in Health and Health Care, for instance, provide a blueprint for individuals and health-care organizations to implement culturally and linguistically appropriate services (Office of Minority Health, n.d.). A 2010 analysis of state pharmacy laws outlines federal requirements for providing pharmacy-related language services to LEP patients through oral interpretation and written translated materials (Spector & Youdelman, 2010). The report also reviews and summarizes state-level laws related to the provision of language services. Because there are significant variations at the state level regarding which services must be provided and how, pharmacists should become familiar with regulations that apply to their practice.

TOOLS FOR COMMUNICATING WITH LEP PATIENTS

Depending on the language needs in the community and the resources available, pharmacies can choose from a variety of tools when communicating with LEP patients. Although not always an option, working with certified interpreters in face-to-face interactions helps to preserve confidentiality, prevent conflicts of interest, and ensure accurate interpretation of the information exchanged. According to a 2002 study by Andrulis, Goodman, and Pryor, more than one-fourth of LEP patients who needed an interpreter but were not provided one—compared with only 2% of those who received one—reported not understanding their medication instructions. The literature clearly demonstrates the benefits of providing competent language services to LEP patients when needed. **Table 7-1** presents a variety of specific communication tools for serving LEP patients and reviews the pros and cons of each.

Table 7-1: Communication Tools for LEP Patients: Pros and Cons

Communication Tools	Pros	Cons
Bilingual pharmacists	• Consistent and dependable • Continuity of service • Valuable for communities with large LEP populations • Direct consultation with patients	• Not always feasible for all LEP communities • Expensive • Cannot adapt easily to new language needs
Bilingual nonclinical staff	• Consistent and dependable • Continuity of service • Valuable for communities with large LEP populations	• Not always feasible for all LEP communities • Cannot provide medication consultation • Expensive • Cannot adapt easily to new language needs
In-person certified interpreters	• Dependable service • Works well for more frequently encountered languages • Ideal for lengthy and complicated conversations, such as a new diagnosis or a complicated treatment plan	• May be expensive, especially for rural areas • Scheduling ahead of time is required
Telephone and/or video interpreters	• Dependable service • Works well for less frequently encountered languages • Scheduling ahead of time is not required	• Not ideal for longer, more complicated conversations • Communication breakdowns possible
Written information in patient's language	• Inexpensive • Can be prepared ahead of time • Can be provided in many languages	• Only feasible for preplanned materials • Not useful for patient consultation • Patients may be illiterate
Ad-hoc interpreters (such as family members)	• No added cost to pharmacy	• Concerns of confidentiality, conflict of interest, interpretation errors, and potential clinical consequences • Not ideal for sensitive health information

PREPARING YOUR PHARMACY FOR LEP PATIENTS

The Language Services Resource Guide for Pharmacists by the National Health Law Program (2010) recommends that community pharmacies take the following step-by-step approach to prepare for serving the needs of LEP patients:

Step 1: Designate responsibility. A full-time staff member in the pharmacy, ideally someone interested and experienced in language services, should assume responsibility in leading the effort.

Step 2: Conduct an analysis of language needs in the community served. Ask your patients about their language needs and preferences, and consult with community organizations to identify languages that should be your priority areas. Ethnic and cultural groups in your area may have associations, community centers, or spiritual or religious organizations that can provide information on the community's demographics. To monitor changing language needs in the patient population, it helps to maintain data on patients' language needs in medical records and management information systems.

Step 3: Identify the available language resources. Gather a list of available resources within the organization and the community. Ideally for the priority languages most prevalent in your community, you will identify resources for different communication needs and scenarios. Consider the communication tools presented earlier.

Step 4: Determine which language services will be provided and how. This may be the most difficult and crucial step in the process. The same LEP patient may do well with written materials in one scenario but need a certified interpreter in another. It is important to evaluate patients' language needs on a case-by-case basis. Another factor is which resources are accessible to the pharmacy.

With constant technology advances, more and more technology-supported tools are becoming available to assist pharmacists in communicating with LEP patients. Some pharmacy chains provide telephonic or Internet-based interpretation to facilitate timely, high-quality communication with LEP patients. Kaiser Permanente pharmacies offer a talking medicine bottle with a microchip on which a pharmacist can record instructions in various languages for patients to play back when needed (National Health Law Program, 2010). Pharmacy professionals should continuously explore and learn more about such tools to improve their services for LEP patients.

LEARN, PRACTICE, AND ASSESS
CASE STUDY EXERCISES

LEARN: Example Patient Dialogues

Directions: Read the following case study. After completing Patient Dialogue One and Patient Dialogue Two, consider the differences between them and answer the questions provided.

PATIENT CASE

A 10-month-old Chinese infant girl was taken to a pediatrician's office by her parents, who do not speak English. The infant was diagnosed with iron-deficiency anemia and prescribed a liquid iron supplement. The parents took the prescription to a local pharmacy that did not provide language services.

PATIENT DIALOGUE ONE

(Mother walks up to the pharmacy counter to fill a new prescription with the infant in her arms and the father standing by her side.)

Pharmacist: Hello. How can I help you?

Mother: (*Hands the prescription to the pharmacist.*)

Pharmacist: (*Takes the prescription.*) Do you want to get this prescription filled? (*Mother and father nod yes.*)

Pharmacist: (*Speaking loudly.*) OKAY, SIT THERE (*pointing to waiting area*).

Pharmacy technician: (*Twenty minutes later: Yells to the waiting area and makes eye contact with the mother holding the infant and pointing to the prescription bag in hand.*) YOUR SCRIPT IS READY! (*Couple walk over to the counter with the infant.*)

Pharmacy technician: (*Talking loud and slow.*) THERE IS NO COPAY. DO YOU HAVE ANY QUESTIONS? (*Mother nods and takes the prescription from the technician; they proceed toward the store exit.*)

Pharmacist technician: (*To the pharmacist.*) They did not have any questions. I think they'll be fine; all of the information is on the bottle and our phone number is there too.

Pharmacist: Sure.

PATIENT DIALOGUE TWO

(Mother walks up to the pharmacy counter to fill a new prescription with the infant in her arms and the father standing by her side.)

Pharmacist: Hello. How can I help you?

Mother: (*Hands the prescription to the pharmacist.*)

Pharmacist: (*Takes the prescription.*) Do you want to get this prescription filled? (*Mother and father nod yes.*)

(The pharmacist reaches for the language sign containing the question "How may I help you" in 10 different languages and shows the sign to the couple. The mother points to the question in Cantonese, a dialect of Chinese. The pharmacist uses the dial-in language service and hands the phone to the mother. The interpreter speaks with the mother; the mother hands the phone back to the pharmacist and heads to the waiting area. The interpreter provides information to the pharmacist to aid in filling the prescription. The pharmacist edits the computer patient profile, updating the language preference to Cantonese. The prescription label and information leaflet are printed in Cantonese. The pharmacist re-phones the interpreter line to have the Cantonese-speaking pharmacist provide instructions on how to administer the infant's prescription. The Cantonese-speaking pharmacist also reminds the pharmacist responsible for the Cantonese patient that new immigrants from some Asian countries may struggle with units of measurement such as milliliters and teaspoons.)

Discussion Questions for the **LEARN** Exercise

1. Consider Dialogue One. What medication errors might have occurred as a result of the lack of communication? What other negative outcomes could have resulted? Consider what the pharmacy and the employees might be liable for if the patient experiences severe adverse outcomes.
2. This text lists several communication tools for serving LEP patients. The pharmacist in Dialogue Two used a telephone interpreter, which might not be available for every patient and every pharmacy setting. Given the patient's family situation, which tool(s) would you try if interpreters were not available?
3. At the end of Dialogue Two, the pharmacist was reminded that, for some LEP patients, units of measurement may be confusing. The mother may not know how to give her infant a teaspoon of medication and mistakenly use a larger spoon. What would you do to explain the different units of measurement to an LEP patient who is learning it for the first time?

LEARN, PRACTICE, AND ASSESS
CASE STUDY EXERCISES

 PRACTICE: Build Your Own Dialogue

Directions: Now it is time to *practice* what you have learned about the topic of this chapter. Reflecting on concepts from this chapter and the patient dialogues in the LEARN exercise, develop your own pharmacist–patient dialogue using the following patient information and guidance questions.

PATIENT CASE

Bithu Desu, a 55-year-old Ethiopian female, presents to a primary care clinic for medication management services with the clinical pharmacist after a recent diagnosis of pancreatic cancer. She has a history of hypothyroidism and type 2 diabetes. The patient speaks limited English and asks to bring her 19-year-old daughter, who is a college student, in the medical room with her. During the interview, the patient is very emotional as she is talking to her daughter about the pancreatic cancer and how much weight she has lost—approximately 30 pounds in the last month without trying. The pharmacist obtains her vital signs and discusses her medications with her daughter in the room to interpret.

- Current medications: Levothyroxine 100 mcg daily, Lantus 40 units SQ QHS

As you plan your dialogue, keep in mind what you have learned about communicating with LEP patients. Use the following questions to help plan and assess your dialogue.

1. An important part of planning a dialogue is setting goals for the conversation. Given the patient's situation, what would you like to accomplish in this dialogue? Be sure to think about both short- and long-term goals. For instance, you may want to first address the patient's emotional state and display empathy and understand more about her pancreatic cancer, but another very important goal might be to communicate your willingness to help, to assess the patient's language needs, and choose the most appropriate communication tool.
2. Which barriers may exist during your patient–pharmacist communication session when using the patient's daughter as an interpreter? Given the patient's disease status and medication regimen, what types of information may likely be misinterpreted when using a layperson as an interpreter?
3. How do you plan to overcome the identified barriers in the previous question during your communication session?

4. How will you confirm that the patient understood the educational
   information provided by you (i.e., verbal and nonverbal cues)?

YOUR DIALOGUE HERE

LEARN, PRACTICE, AND ASSESS
CASE STUDY EXERCISES

☐ ASSESS: Build Your Own Dialogue

Directions: Now it is time to *assess* what you have learned about the topic of this chapter. In this exercise, no guidance questions are provided. Reflect on what you have learned from the LEARN and PRACTICE exercises, and develop your own pharmacist–patient dialogue using the following patient information.

PATIENT CASE

Luis Perez is a 57-year-old postmenopausal female from Mexico. She lives with her daughter, son-in-law, and grandchildren, and she speaks limited English. Ms. Perez was diagnosed with diabetes 6 months ago and started on an oral diabetes medication. Ms. Perez is being seen in the clinic today for diabetes management and follow up and brings her grandson in to help translate.

- Current medications: Metformin 1000 mg 1 tablet by mouth BID (type 2 DM)

Ms. Perez believes that her diabetes is caused by the spirit of her ancestors who are angry that she left Mexico. She recently visited a *curandera* (traditional healer) who gave her some herbs to take, including garlic. She stopped taking the Metformin and started the herbs 2 weeks ago because she began losing her hair and having diarrhea and often felt nauseous.

YOUR DIALOGUE HERE

DISCUSSION QUESTIONS

1. Which language services are you aware of that exist in your hospital, clinic, and/or community pharmacy setting?
2. Which barriers may exist for pharmacists who wish to provide more language services in the community pharmacy setting?
3. Consider the area that you serve or hope to serve. How has the community's language needs changed over the years? How might they change in the coming decades? In what ways can healthcare professionals keep up with the population's evolving language needs due to immigration and other population changes?
4. Some healthcare professionals do not see the value of providing language services to immigrants because "they chose to come here and should have learned the language." This view exists in the community as well. How would you respond to someone with this perspective?
5. This text discusses the steps needed to prepare a community pharmacy for LEP patients. Consider the pharmacy setting you plan to work at and the community you will serve. How feasible are these steps?

REFERENCES

Agency for Healthcare Research and Quality. (2012). *Improving patient safety systems for patients with limited English proficiency: A guide for hospitals.* Rockville, MD: Author.

Andrulis, D., Goodman, N., & Pryor, C. (2002). *What a difference an interpreter can make: Health care experiences of uninsured with limited English proficiency.* Boston, MA: The Access Project.

National Health Law Program. (2010). *Language services resource guide for pharmacists.* Washington, DC: Author.

Office of Minority Health, U.S. Department of Health and Human Services. (n.d.). *CLAS and the CLAS standards.* Retrieved from https://www.thinkculturalhealth.hhs.gov/content/clas.asp

Spector, S. L., & Youdelman, M. (2010). *Analysis of state pharmacy laws: Impact of pharmacy laws on the provision of language services.* Washington, DC: National Health Law Program.

USA.gov. (2013). *Learn about life in the United States.* Retrieved from https://www.usa.gov/life-in-the-us#item-36017

U.S. Census Bureau. (2013, August 6). *New Census Bureau interactive map shows languages spoken in America* [News release]. Retrieved from http://www.census.gov/newsroom/releases/archives/education/cb13-143.html

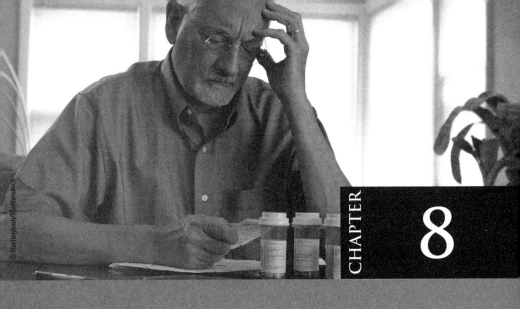

COMMUNICATING WITH PATIENTS WITH LOW HEALTH LITERACY

LEARNING OBJECTIVES

At the end of this chapter, students should be able to:

▸ Recognize low health literacy as a public health problem.

▸ Recognize the common myths related to health literacy.

▸ Apply various tools to address low health literacy in the context of pharmacist–patient communication.

KEY TERMS

Health literacy

The 2010 Patient Protection and Affordable Care Act defines health literacy as the degree to which individuals have the capacity to obtain, process, and understand basic health information and services needed to make appropriate health decisions (Centers for Disease Control and Prevention, 2015). For pharmacy patients, health literacy skills include understanding why a medication is prescribed, reading medication labels, understanding side effects, being able to calculate dosage, and managing multiple medications. Given that communication with a pharmacist in regard to medication instructions is often the last opportunity to ensure proper understanding and prevent medication error, pharmacists play a crucial role in assisting patients with limited health literacy.

FACTS ABOUT HEALTH LITERACY

Individuals' health literacy skills are mediated by their education, culture, and language, among other factors. According to the Health Resources and Services Administration (n.d.), low health literacy is more prevalent among older adults, minority populations, individuals with limited education, individuals with low socioeconomic status, and medically underserved people. As you reflect on how low health literacy may affect the patient populations you serve, consider the following facts about health literacy in the United States:

- Low health literacy costs the U.S. economy between $106 billion and $236 billion annually (University of Connecticut, 2007).
- Only 12% of U.S. adults have proficient health literacy (e.g., can interpret the prescription label correctly) (U.S. Department of Health and Human Services, n.d.).
- Over a third of U.S. adults—77 million people—would have difficulty with common health tasks, such as following directions on a medication label or adhering to a childhood immunization schedule using a standard chart (U.S. Department of Health and Human Services, 2008).
- Low health literacy affects adults in all racial and ethnic groups, but not equally. The proportion of adults with basic or below basic health literacy ranges from 28% of white adults to 65% of Hispanic adults (U.S. Department of Health and Human Services, 2008).
- One study found that most patients remember about 40% to 50% of what they hear in the doctor's office but many do not ask for clarification (Kessels, 2003).
- Literacy skills are a stronger predictor of an individual's health status than age, income, employment status, education level, or racial/ethnic group (Weiss, 2003).

Pharmacy professionals must address low health literacy in order to help their patients achieve optimum care through medication treatment. Medication errors are more likely among patients with limited health literacy, as they often misinterpret the prescription label information and auxiliary labels. Given that pharmacists are the most accessible healthcare providers in the community, they also have more opportunities to understand patients' struggles with health literacy and provide assistance.

MYTHS ABOUT HEALTH LITERACY

- *Myth*: "I serve a community that is pretty affluent; most of my patients are educated and work full time. Surely they do not have a problem reading or doing math."
  Fact: A high level of education or being otherwise highly functional in life does not always equal a high level of health literacy. Imagine that a highly educated individual just received a new diagnosis of a life-changing disease and needs to start a complicated medication regimen. Regardless of education and socioeconomic status, the typical patient will feel overwhelmed with the information and with the decision he or she has to make. Educating the patient and ensuring proper understanding is important.
- *Myth*: "I always ask my patients whether they have any questions about the medication. If patients are confused, they will speak up and ask for clarification."
  Fact: Low health literacy is not easily recognized. Patients with low health literacy often are very good at masking their challenges and may have developed well-practiced coping mechanisms over the years. For instance, a patient may refuse to read information provided for them, using the excuse that they do not have their glasses, or they want to fill out forms later. Instead of asking questions at the pharmacy, they may ask friends or family members for help, which could lead to misunderstanding.
- *Myth*: "If I ask my patients to ask more questions, it'll take up time that I already do not have. Plus, there is usually a line of patients waiting; I simply cannot afford to spend more time with a patient than I have to."
  Fact: Working with patients with limited health literacy may require longer consultation time, especially in initial conversations when a patient may still be uncomfortable or avoidant. However, investing those extra minutes not only ensures that the patient has a proper understanding of why he or she is taking the medication and how, but more important, establishes a line of trust and open communication between you and the patient. As a result, the patient is more likely to trust you with future questions. Investing in health literacy-related patient needs reduces medication error, improves patient compliance, and leads to better patient outcomes in the long run.

HEALTH LITERACY INFLUENCES HEALTH

Low health literacy negatively influences health outcomes. The U.S. Department of Health and Human Services (n.d.) identified four reasons why health information is difficult to use and understand:

1. Complexity of the information presentation
2. Use of unfamiliar scientific and medical jargon
3. Demands of navigating the healthcare system, including locating providers and services and filling out forms
4. Difficulty that people of all literacy levels have in understanding information when confronted with a stressful or unfamiliar health situation that affects them or their loved ones

All four reasons could complicate communication between pharmacists and their patients, but they also suggest specific ways that pharmacists can help patients with low health literacy: by presenting medication-related information in a clear, easy-to-understand format, by assisting patients in navigating the insurance system, and so on.

HEALTH LITERACY TOOLS FOR PHARMACISTS

There are a variety of tools available that pharmacists can use to help patients with low health literacy. For instance, the Agency for Healthcare Research and Quality (2014) developed the following health literacy tools for pharmacists:

- Conduct a *Pharmacy Health Literacy Assessment* to see how well your pharmacy is set up to serve patients with limited health literacy. With this tool, a pharmacy can assess whether its patient needs, affected by various levels of health literacy, are being met, identify potential barriers that may create challenges for their patients with limited health literacy skills, and identify strategies to improve communication with these patients.
- Provide low health literacy patients with *tools to educate and empower* them. For instance, keeping track of multiple medications can be particularly challenging for patients with low health literacy. Providing them with custom-designed pill cards, which contain simple, visual information about the medications, can be beneficial for patients.
- Practice *clear communication* both orally and in written materials. Medical terminology can make conversations and written materials about health issues overwhelming for the patient. When explaining a medical issue or medication to a patient, be sure to practice principles of clear communication, or plain-language communication, by using familiar, shorter words, using the active voice whenever possible, and avoiding jargon.
- Use the *teach-back method* to ensure understanding. After explaining the information, ask the patient to restate it in his or her own words. If the patient's understanding is inaccurate or incomplete, the pharmacist can then repeat the information or present it differently. This method has

been shown to effectively increase patient adherence to treatment plans and is recommended by the National Quality Forum (2009) as a top patient safety practice.

- Emphasize *one to three key points* during the oral consultation, and provide additional informational materials that are accessible to the patient and family members. With this technique, the pharmacist helps the patient prioritize the information that is most relevant to adherence.

Low health literacy is a challenge faced by all healthcare professionals, and pharmacists have a critical role to play as they act as the *last line of defense* in recognizing patients who may struggle with low health literacy and preventing adverse outcomes such as medication errors or low adherence.

LEARN, PRACTICE, AND ASSESS
CASE STUDY EXERCISES

● **LEARN:** Example Patient Dialogues

Directions: Read the following case study. After completing Patient Dialogue One and Patient Dialogue Two, consider the differences between them and answer the questions provided.

PATIENT CASE

Cathy Myers, a well-dressed 67-year-old Caucasian female, presents to her community pharmacy in the high-end part of town, where she has been going for the past 11 years. She often comes into the pharmacy with her grandson and usually is in a rush to get her prescription and leave. She was recently diagnosed with chronic obstructive pulmonary disease (COPD) and was instructed by her physician to obtain an influenza and pneumococcal vaccination at her local pharmacy, instead of at her doctor's office. She is a homemaker who homeschooled her kids and is now helping to take care of her 4-year-old grandson 3 days a week.

- Past medical history:
  - COPD (diagnosed 1 month ago)
  - Hypertension x 20 years
  - Osteoporosis x 1 year
  - Postmenopausal x 15 years

- Current medications:
  - HCTZ 25 mg 1 tablet po daily
  - Boniva 150 mg 1 tablet po monthly
  - Spiriva 18 mg 1 inhalation po daily
  - Albuterol inhaler prn SOB

PATIENT DIALOGUE ONE

Pharmacist: Hello, Mrs. Myers. Hi there, Caleb. How was your Thanksgiving?

Patient: Hi, Janet. We had a great time! All of my kids were able to come home this year. We had about 20 people over, including all of the grandkids and spouses. It was the first time everyone has been home in about 3 years. (*Caleb starts walking toward the OTC aisles picking up medications.*) Caleb, come back over here.

Pharmacist: That's great! How can I help you today?

Patient: My doctor told me that I can start to get my flu shot done here. I didn't know you all can give flu shots now.

Pharmacist: Yes, we can! I would be glad to give you your flu shot today, and you should also receive another vaccine called the *pneumococcal vaccine* because of your recent COPD diagnosis. I just need you to fill out this paperwork (*hands the vaccination form on a clipboard to the patient*) and bring it back to me when you are finished and I can give you your shot right away.

Patient: Oh yes, my doctor did mention the pneumococcal vaccine too, so that would be great. Do I have to fill out the form right now before you can give me the shots? (*Looks concerned.*)

Pharmacist: Yes, it will only take a few minutes and you can fill it out there (*pointing*) in the waiting area.

Patient: Okay. (*The patient walks over to the waiting area still looking concerned; the pharmacist gets back to work.*)

(The patient returns to the consultation window 2 minutes later and hands the vaccination form to the pharmacist. The pharmacist looks at the form and notices it only has her name filled in.)

Patient: Janet, I will have to come back later with my husband because Caleb is getting restless and I was not able to fill out the form, plus I forgot my glasses.

Pharmacist: No problem, Mrs. Myers. We will see you later. Have a great day.

PATIENT DIALOGUE TWO

Pharmacist: Hello, how can I help you?

Patient: Hi. Where's Janet? Are you the new pharmacist? (*Caleb, the patient's grandson, starts walking toward the OTC aisles picking up medications.*) Caleb, come back over here.

Pharmacist: Janet is off today. I am the new pharmacist. Nice to meet you.

Patient: I'm Mrs. Myers, nice to meet you. My doctor sent me here to get my flu shot. I didn't know you all can give flu shots now.

Pharmacist: Yes, we can! I would be glad to give you your flu shot today, and you should also receive another vaccine called the *pneumococcal vaccine* because of your recent COPD diagnosis. I just need you to fill out this paperwork (*hands the vaccination form on a clipboard to the patient*) and bring it back to me when you are finished and I can give you your shot right away.

Patient: Oh yes, my doctor did mention the pneumococcal vaccine too, so that would be great. Do I have to fill out the form right now before you can give me the shots? (*Looks concerned.*)

Pharmacist: (*The pharmacist notices Mrs. Myers's concerned look.*) Yes, it will only take a few minutes. Would you like for either myself or my technician to come out and help you?

Patient: That would be great, but I know that you are busy so I can just come back later with my husband. Caleb is getting restless and I left my reading glasses at home.

Pharmacist: (*The pharmacist picks up on the patient's cues of leaving her glasses at home and wanting to get help from her husband when filling out the vaccination form.*) We would be glad to help you. Please let me get my technician. She will meet you in the waiting area and will bring some coloring books to occupy Caleb while you fill out the forms.

Patient: Oh, that would be great. I really appreciate your taking the time to help me; it really means a lot. I have a hard time understanding all of these medical forms, so it would be wonderful to get her help.

Pharmacist: We are glad to help! Please don't ever hesitate to ask one of us any questions you may have about your medicines because that's what we are here for. Amy will be over shortly. (*Turns to the technician.*) Please go out to the waiting area and help Mrs. Myers fill out her immunization forms.

Discussion Questions for the **LEARN** Exercise

1. Which signs did Mrs. Meyers display that may suggest she could be trying to hide her low health literacy levels? Consider your own practice or ask someone who has practiced. Which common signs do patients often display that may suggest they are struggling with low literacy or low health literacy?

2. The pharmacist in Dialogue One missed the opportunity to identify and assist a patient with possible low health literacy. Knowing the potential consequences of low health literacy, how do you plan to prevent making the same mistake?

3. Consider the various tools reviewed in this chapter for assisting patients with low health literacy. How could these tools be used to assist Mrs. Meyers if she needs help understanding the instruction of a new medication or learn how to measure and monitor her blood sugar level?

4. This text discusses several myths, which might cause a pharmacist to miss the opportunity to identify and help a patient with low literacy or low health literacy. Consider the demographic profile of Mrs. Meyers. What about her might explain why the pharmacist in Dialogue One failed to recognize her struggle with low health literacy? What other myths can you think of that may exist regarding health literacy?

LEARN, PRACTICE, AND ASSESS
CASE STUDY EXERCISES

▲ PRACTICE: Build Your Own Dialogue

Directions: Now it is time to *practice* what you have learned about the topic of this chapter. Reflecting on concepts from this chapter and the patient dialogues in the LEARN exercise, develop your own pharmacist–patient dialogue using the following patient information and guidance questions.

PATIENT CASE

A 62-year-old African-American female presents to a free health clinic to order medication refills from a patient assistance program. She needs to reorder Benicar HCT 40/12.5 mg, Crestor 10 mg, and Lantus insulin 30 units. She is given some forms to complete for the patient assistance program and states that she has forgotten her glasses. She would like to take the forms home and bring them back the next day. The pharmacist comes into the medicine room to speak with the patient, who asks the pharmacist if she has time to talk about her medications. The pharmacist is happy to speak with her. The patient asks the pharmacist to help her fill out the patient assistance forms.

As you plan your dialogue, keep in mind what you have learned about communicating with low health literacy patients. Use the following questions to help plan and assess your dialogue.

1. An important part of planning a dialogue is setting goals for the conversation. Given the patient's situation, what would you like to accomplish in this dialogue? Be sure to think about both short- and long-term goals. For instance, you may want to inquire about her medication adherence, and find out whether she understands how to take her medications and whether she has any problems she wants to discuss. However, an important long-term communication goal may be to help her become more comfortable with you, so that you two can openly discuss difficult topics, such as struggles with health literacy.

2. For patients with low health literacy, it is important to recognize the potential signs because patients may not be willing to directly share their misunderstanding of health information or their inability to read. In your dialogue, be sure to plan verbal and nonverbal strategies to address this.

3. The patient seems comfortable asking the pharmacist for help with her medications. As a pharmacist, what can you do to encourage low health literacy patients to seek help from you? How can you make the patient feel more comfortable?

4. There are a variety of health literacy tools for pharmacists to use when educating patients. Which specific tools do you plan to use to educate and empower the low health literacy patient?
5. How will you ensure that the patient understands the information you provide?

YOUR DIALOGUE HERE

LEARN, PRACTICE, AND ASSESS
CASE STUDY EXERCISES

ASSESS: Build Your Own Dialogue

Directions: Now it is time to *assess* what you have learned about the topic of this chapter. In this exercise, no guidance questions are provided. Reflect on what you have learned from the LEARN and PRACTICE exercises, and develop your own pharmacist–patient dialogue using the following patient information.

PATIENT CASE

A mother comes to your pharmacy complaining that she has been giving her son medicine for his ear infection for the past 5 days and he seems to be getting fussier and pulling at his ear instead of getting better. You ask the mother to show you how she is administering the antibiotic (Amoxicillin) to her son using a dropper, and she demonstrates putting it in his ear.

YOUR DIALOGUE HERE

DISCUSSION QUESTIONS

1. In what ways might new technologies, such as hand-held devices, be used to assist patients with low health literacy?
2. Patients with low literacy levels, or who struggle with understanding what you are saying, may manage to mask their struggles to avoid talking about their issues. How can you make a patient feel more comfortable with needing extra assistance with health-related information? How would you bring up the issue without embarrassing or offending the patient?
3. As stated in this text, most patients remember no more than half of what they hear at the doctor's office and yet they do not ask for clarification. Therefore, some argue that pharmacy professionals are the last line of defense when it comes to identifying patients with low health literacy and helping them before a costly mistake occurs when they go home. Do you agree? What role should a pharmacist play, as a member of the healthcare team, in addressing the needs of low health literacy patients?

REFERENCES

Agency for Healthcare Research and Quality. (2014). *AHRQ health literacy tools for use in pharmacies*. Retrieved from http://www.ahrq.gov/professionals /quality-patient-safety/pharmhealthlit/tools.html

Centers for Disease Control and Prevention. (2015). *Learn about health literacy*. Retrieved from http://www.cdc.gov/healthliteracy/Learn/index.html

Health Resources and Services Administration. (n.d.). *About health literacy*. Retrieved from http://www.hrsa.gov/publichealth/healthliteracy/healthlitabout.html

Kessels, R. P. C. (2003). Patients' memory for medical information. *Journal of the Royal Society of Medicine, 96*(5), 219–222.

National Quality Forum. (2009). *Safe practices for better healthcare—2009 update*. Retrieved from http://www.qualityforum.org/Publications/2009/03 /Safe_Practices_for_Better _Healthcare%E2%80%932009_Update.aspx

University of Connecticut. (2007, October 12). *New report estimates cost of low health literacy between $106 – $236 billion annually* [News release]. Retrieved from http://www.prnewswire.com/news-releases/new-report-estimates-cost-of-low -health-literacy-between-106–236-billion-annually-58522037.html

U.S. Department of Health and Human Services. (2008). *America's health literacy: Why we need accessible health information*. Retrieved from http://www.health.gov /communication /literacy/issuebrief/

U.S. Department of Health and Human Services. (n.d.). *Quick guide to health literacy*. Retrieved from http://www.health.gov/communication/literacy/quickguide /factsbasic.htm

Weiss, B. D. (2003). *Health literacy: A manual for clinicians*. Chicago, IL: American Medical Association Foundation and American Medical Association.

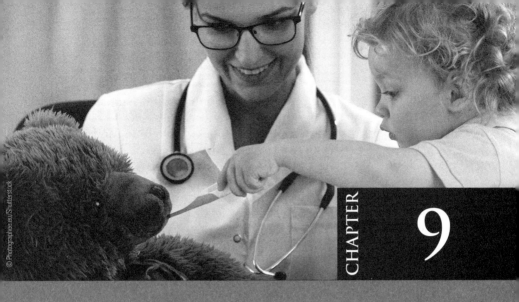

COMMUNICATING WITH YOUNG PATIENTS

LEARNING OBJECTIVES

At the end of this chapter, students should be able to:

▸ Recognize the pharmacist's role and responsibilities in serving the needs, including the communication needs, of young patients.

▸ Discuss the different cognitive developmental stages of children and the effects on patient communication.

▸ Identify principles and strategies useful for communicating with young patients.

▸ Generate communication strategies to provide counseling to young patients.

Effective verbal and written communication skills for ensuring medication adherence, patient safety, and optimal outcomes is vital. Many effective communication strategies developed for adults also apply to children. However, children often require a different approach based on their developmental stages as well as the child–caregiver interaction.

In 1999, the U.S. Pharmacopeia developed the position statement "Ten Guiding Principles for Teaching Children and Adolescents About Medicines," which supports the right of children to receive information and direct communication about medicines (Bush, Ozias, Walson, & Ward, 1999). The National Council on Patient Information and Education (2007) also emphasizes the importance of direct communication between pharmacists and children.

Despite these recommendations, children often do not receive counseling about their medications from physicians or pharmacists. Nilaward, Mason, and Newton (2005) conducted a study with 460 community pharmacists to determine the daily percentage of children to whom the pharmacists talked directly about medications. On average, pharmacists reported communicating about medications with 20.7% of children compared to 57% of adults. The factors significantly influencing frequency of communication included the experience one had as a pharmacy student preceptor and the pharmacy prescription volume. Pharmacists provided more information to parents than to children and more medication information to older children than to younger children. When children of all ages did receive medication information, they were likely to be comforted and provided information about the medicine's taste. This low incidence of pediatric medication education may be related to a lack of comfort among healthcare providers due to limited experience providing health information to children. Because the majority of pharmacists will work with pediatric patients at some point in their careers, it is important to develop communication skills for delivering age-appropriate information and building a trusting patient–provider relationship with this unique patient population.

COGNITIVE DEVELOPMENT

To effectively communicate with children, the information must be presented at a level appropriate for their comprehension. The Federal Drug Administration, for instance, recommends that parents and guardians provide their children age-appropriate information on how to use medication safely (2013). Similarly, pharmacy professionals ought to understand the unique needs of children at each age level. Piaget (1932) proposed four stages of cognitive development for children: sensorimotor, preoperational, concrete operational, and formal operational. **Table 9-1** details the features and level of information appropriate for medication counseling at each stage (Sleath, Bush, & Pradel, 2003). Not all children will progress through the stages at the same rate; therefore, it is important to assess each patient's developmental stage through the use of open-ended questions. Also, this method of staging does not apply to children with learning disabilities or disease states that may impair cognitive development.

Table 9-1: Piaget's Cognitive Developmental Stages and the Effects on Medication Counseling

Approximate Age (years)	Developmental Stage	Features	Medication Counseling
0–2	Sensorimotor	• Minimal connection to objects outside the self	Learning about medications is not possible (counseling is therefore provided to the caregiver).
2–7	Preoperational	• One aspect of a situation considered • Limited attention span	Pharmacists can provide education on medications; however, the amount of information presented must be limited (why it is important to take the medication, dosage forms and how to take the medication, adverse effects, etc.).
7–11	Concrete operational	• Able to focus on multiple factors at one time • Development of problem-solving skills	Pharmacists can provide education in such areas as how drugs work, where they "go" in the body, why there are different drugs for different illnesses, adverse effects, and the importance of medication adherence.
≥ 12	Formal operational	• Capable of hypothetical and abstract thinking • Able to reason logically	Pharmacists can provide education in such areas as the differences between prescription and nonprescription medications, the need for taking medications on particular schedules, the potential for drug interactions, the difference between brand and generic drugs, how to select an appropriate nonprescription medication, a drug's purpose, adverse effects, and the importance of medication adherence.

GENERAL COMMUNICATION PRINCIPLES AND ESTABLISHING RAPPORT WITH CHILDREN

Children and adolescents may be hesitant to talk with adults who are unfamiliar to them. It is important to approach the conversation in a manner that will make the patient feel comfortable and allow trust to develop. Nonverbal communication is a key component when interacting with children. Pharmacists talking with children should sit at or below children's eye level and be cognizant of their facial expressions, tone of voice, and gestures (Sleath et al., 2003). You may even want to kneel down to obtain eye contact. Other general recommendations for communicating with children include the following:

- Provide your full attention.
- Remain calm and nonjudgmental.
- Begin the conversation by discussing something of interest to the child.
- Give them plenty of time to respond to questions.
- Allow them adequate time to express concerns and ask questions.
- Listen attentively and repeat to ensure understanding.
- Allow them to participate in making decisions about their medications.

Specific open-ended questions should be utilized when obtaining information from the child or adolescent. Immediate follow-up with more direct, closed-ended questions is appropriate. It is essential to remember that children often respond to adults with the answer they expect will please the adult. Reassuring the child or adolescent that providing the honest response is acceptable and preferred may be necessary.

UNIQUE CHALLENGES OF COMMUNICATING WITH CAREGIVERS OF YOUNG PATIENTS

While it is essential that the discussion be directed toward the pediatric patient if age appropriate, it is also important to include the caregiver. This is accomplished by first communicating with the child, addressing his or her questions and concerns, and then giving attention to the caregiver's questions and concerns. When providing education on medications, this may also be done as a group, signifying a team effort in which everyone is working together to improve the health of the patient, including the caregiver.

Another factor to be cognizant of with caregiver communication is the multitude of emotions that may be present. Caregivers are often more fearful of the child's health than they would be of their own. The caregiver may also feel guilt, typically unwarranted, as a result of the child's poor health. Either of these emotions can cause them to react in abnormal ways. It is important as the health provider to remain calm and offer reassurance as appropriate. Utilizing effective verbal and nonverbal communication skills can help alleviate the tension and provide better consultation with the caregiver.

Children and adolescents are important consumers of pharmaceutical care who require a unique approach to medication counseling. It is important to cater to the pediatric patient as best as possible. For example, most liquid medications include a variety of more palatable flavors such as grape, cherry, or bubble gum. Providing this option can not only enhance medication adherence for pediatric patients but also benefit the patient–provider relationship through effective patient accommodation. In addition, pharmacists can inquire if the patient prefers liquid or pill medications. It is important not to assume that an older child is able to swallow a pill. It is ideal to empower pediatric patients to make choices when communicating about their medications. Pharmacists can play an essential role in effective communication with children, adolescents, and their caregivers. With practice, this can be a rewarding experience that positively influences medication adherence, patient safety, and optimal outcomes in this vulnerable patient population.

LEARN, PRACTICE, AND ASSESS
CASE STUDY EXERCISES

 LEARN: Example Patient Dialogues

Directions: Read the following case study. After completing Patient Dialogue One and Patient Dialogue Two, consider the differences between them and answer the questions provided.

PATIENT CASE

A 9-year-old female with mother-to-child transmitted HIV presents to the clinic for a follow-up appointment with her mother. Based on suboptimal laboratory values (elevated viral load, below-goal CD4 count), the medical team is concerned about medication adherence. Her current medication regimen includes the following:

* Kaletra 100/25 mg tablet: 3 tablets by mouth every 12 hours
* Lamivudine 100 mg tablet: 1 tablet by mouth every 12 hours
* Zidovudine 100 mg capsule: 2 capsules by mouth every 12 hours

Upon entering the patient's room, the patient is in no acute distress but appears distracted as she plays a game on her iPad. Her mother appears slightly tense but approachable.

PATIENT DIALOGUE ONE

Pharmacist: Hello, Ms. Smith. I am the clinical pharmacist for the pediatric HIV clinic, and I am here to talk to you about Abby's medications.

Patient's caregiver: Okay.

(The patient continues to play her game without looking up.)

Pharmacist: How is Abby doing with her medications? Any issues or side effects?

Patient's caregiver: She doesn't have any side effects with them, but it is a struggle to get her to take every dose. It takes 2 hours to get her to take the doses. I don't have time for that in the mornings before school and work. I don't know what else to do. I've tried everything. (*The patient's mother appears stressed and tense as she grips her chair.*)

Pharmacist: How many doses has she missed in the last month?

Patient's caregiver: Um, I'm not sure. Maybe three or four doses each week. I'm just so tired of fighting with her to take her medications.

Pharmacist: I understand that it can be difficult, but it is very important that she take every dose. To get her laboratory values to the goal levels, she needs to receive every dose.

Patient's caregiver: I understand. (*The patient's mother appears guilty and discouraged and looks down at her hands.*)

PATIENT DIALOGUE TWO

Pharmacist: Hello, Ms. Smith. I am the clinical pharmacist for the pediatric HIV clinic. Hi, Abby. How are you today? Is this a new game?

Patient's caregiver: Hello.

Patient: (*Looks up from her handheld game.*) I'm good. Yes, I got this from my grandparents for my birthday last week.

Pharmacist: (*The pharmacist sits in a chair beside the patient.*) That's awesome! I just bought my niece that same game for her birthday last month. I wanted to talk to you about your medications. Do you mind pausing your game for a few minutes?

Patient: Sure (*pauses the game and sets it aside; appears comfortable and open to conversation*).

Pharmacist: Abby, how is it going with your medications? Are you having any issues or side effects?

Patient: Good. No issues.

Patient's caregiver: She doesn't have any side effects with them, but it is a struggle to get her to take every dose. It takes 2 hours to get her to take the doses. I don't have time for that in the mornings before school and work. I don't know what else to do. I've tried everything. (*The patient's mother appears stressed and tense as she grips her chair.*)

Pharmacist: (*Looking at the patient's mother.*) It sounds like she tolerates the medications but has issues taking them. (*Looking at the patient who is now looking at the floor.*) Abby, can you explain what makes it difficult to take the medications?

Patient: I just don't like taking medicine. Sometimes my stomach hurts when I'm on the bus to school after taking the medications.

Patient's caregiver: (*Looking at the patient.*) You never told me that.

Pharmacist: These medications can upset your stomach if taken without food. I can understand why that would make you hesitant to take the medications. Do you eat breakfast at home or at school?

Patient: Sometimes I eat breakfast at home, but most of the time I eat breakfast at school.

Patient's caregiver: The mornings are so crazy trying to get everyone ready for school and work. We don't have time to sit down for breakfast, and they provide it at school.

Pharmacist: (*Looking at the patient's mother.*) That is totally understandable. Would it be possible for Abby to take a breakfast bar or something with her to eat on the bus so that the medicine doesn't upset her stomach?

Patient's caregiver: We could do that.

Pharmacist: Abby, do you have a favorite breakfast bar or something that you could have in your backpack to eat on the bus?

Patient: I like granola bars.

Pharmacist: Excellent! This should help prevent the stomachaches from the medication. If you are still having stomachaches, I need you to tell your mother so she can let us know. Can you do that for me?

Patient: I can do that.

Pharmacist: Great! It is very important that you take care of your body; you only have one body, you know (*smiles*). It is also important to tell your mother and me if you have any other problems with your medications in the future. We are here to work together with you.

Patient: Okay, I will.

Discussion Questions for the **LEARN** Exercise

1. Compare and discuss how the pharmacist interacted with the patient in the two dialogues. Which verbal and nonverbal communication strategies did the pharmacist in Dialogue Two use to engage with the patient?
2. The pharmacist in Dialogue Two successfully communicated with the patient and helped figure out the real reason behind her nonadherence. In addition to this immediate benefit, what long-term benefits might this successful communication bring to the pharmacist–patient relationship?
3. The patient in the case study is 9 years old. Do you think the pharmacist in Dialogue Two communicated appropriately given the patient's age? If the patient was 6 years old, or 14 years old, how might the communication challenges and dynamics change?

LEARN, PRACTICE, AND ASSESS
CASE STUDY EXERCISES

▲ PRACTICE: Build Your Own Dialogue

Directions: Now it is time to *practice* what you have learned about the topic of this chapter. Reflecting on concepts from this chapter and the patient dialogues in the LEARN exercise, develop your own pharmacist–patient dialogue using the following patient information and guidance questions.

PATIENT CASE

A 12-year-old female has just been diagnosed with type 1 diabetes. She is started on Humulin 70/30 insulin 10 units twice daily. The patient and her parents are confused and do not know what to expect. They arrive at the diabetes clinic for a basic diabetes education class by the diabetes educator who is a pharmacist. The patient has a lot of questions about being able to play with her friends and going to school while taking the injections daily. The patient and her parents display verbal and nonverbal signs of worry.

As you plan your dialogue, keep in mind what you have learned about communicating with young patients. Use the following questions to help plan and assess your dialogue.

1. An important part of planning a dialogue is setting goals for the conversation. Given the patient's and family's situation, what would you like to accomplish in this dialogue? Be sure to think about both short- and long-term goals. For instance, you may want to address the patients' and parents' immediate concerns and worries, while at the same time making an effort toward building a trusting relationship as a long-term goal.
2. Which potential barriers to communication with the young patient may exist? Which communication barriers may exist with the caregivers? How do you plan to overcome those barriers?
3. It is very important to gain rapport with children during pharmacy communication sessions. This will also help you to gain rapport with the parents. What specific ways will you gain rapport with the patient and her family?
4. When communicating with young patients, it is important to address the patient's concerns first and then address the caregiver's concerns. It is also important not to provide too much verbal information during a single communication session. Develop an outline of the information you want to cover during this session and the order of the information.

5. Discussing a new health diagnosis with anyone, especially a child, can be overwhelming. How will you ensure that both the patient and the parents understand the information you provide during this communication session?

YOUR DIALOGUE HERE

LEARN, PRACTICE, AND ASSESS
CASE STUDY EXERCISES

 ASSESS: Build Your Own Dialogue

Directions: Now it is time to *assess* what you have learned about the topic of this chapter. In this exercise, no guidance questions are provided. Reflect on what you have learned from the LEARN and PRACTICE exercises, and develop your own pharmacist–patient dialogue using the following patient information.

PATIENT CASE

A 4-year-old male and his father present to your community pharmacy with the following prescriptions:

- Albuterol inhaler 1 to 2 puffs with spacer q4h prn difficulty breathing
- Orapred (prednisolone) 15 mg/5 ml 2 teaspoonful (10 ml) po daily x 5 days

The father appears anxious and slightly stressed. He explains that they were just released from the emergency room after being treated for an "asthma attack" and that he has never used these medications before. The patient appears calm but clings to his father and holds his teddy bear tightly under his arm.

YOUR DIALOGUE HERE

DISCUSSION QUESTIONS

1. Consider your personal and professional experiences as well as your background. What experiences or qualities do you think you have that may prepare you for communicating with young patients?
2. Which strategies do you plan to utilize when educating children and their caregivers about medications?
3. This text discusses the different stages of cognitive development that pharmacists should consider while working with pediatric patients. What about their emotional state? Their social lives? Discuss how these factors might affect a pharmacist's communication with pediatric patients.
4. Children currently have access to a multitude of health information via the Internet. In what ways could this create challenges for healthcare professionals as they talk to children about medications? In what ways might pharmacists use this information to their advantage while serving pediatric patients?

REFERENCES

Bush, P. J., Ozias, J. M., Walson, P. D., & Ward, R. M. (1999). Ten guiding principles for teaching children and adolescents about medicines. *Clinical Therapeutics, 21*(7), 1280–1284.

Condren, M. (2013). Communicating with children, adolescents, and their caregivers. In S. Benavides & M. C. Nahata (Eds.), *Pediatric pharmacotherapy* (pp. 61–66). Lenexa, KS: American College of Clinical Pharmacy.

FDA. (2013). As they grow: Teaching your children how to use medicines safely. Accessed on July 21, 2015 at http://www.fda.gov/Drugs/ResourcesForYou /Consumers/BuyingUsingMedicineSafely/UnderstandingOver-the- CounterMedicines/ucm094876.htm

National Council of Patient Information and Education. (2007). *Enhancing prescription medicine adherence: A national action plan.* Rockville, MD: Author.

Nilaward, W., Mason, H. L., & Newton, G. D. (2005). Community pharmacist-child medication communication: Magnitude, influences, and content. *Journal of the American Pharmacists Association, 45*(3), 354–362.

Piaget, J. (1932). *The moral judgment of the child.* New York, NY: Harcourt, Brace & World.

Sleath, B., Bush, P. J., & Pradel, F. G. (2003). Communicating with children about medicines: A pharmacist's perspective. *American Journal of Health-System Pharmacy, 60*(6), 604–607.

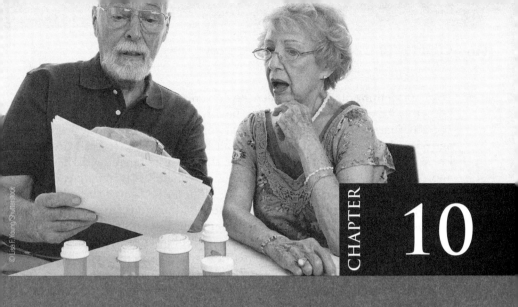

CHAPTER 10

COMMUNICATING WITH OLDER PATIENTS

LEARNING OBJECTIVES

At the end of this chapter, students should be able to:

▸ Recognize the pharmacist's role and responsibilities in serving the needs, including the communication needs, of older patients.

▸ Recognize various stereotypes related to aging.

▸ Discuss how cognitive impairment associated with aging may affect pharmacist–patient communication.

▸ Generate strategies useful for communicating with older patients.

The number of adults over the age of 65 in the United States continues to grow at a rapid rate and is expected to more than double between the years 2000 and 2030, according to a 2014 report by the Administration on Aging. Compared to other age groups, adults in this category carry a heavier burden of chronic illness, make more visits to physicians, and utilize more prescription medications on an annual basis. In addition, 35% of men and 38% of women aged 65 and over have some level of disability or limitations in activity (i.e., difficulty in hearing, vision, cognition, ambulation, self-care, or independent living). The ability to communicate effectively with older adults regarding their health care will become ever more important as the number of Americans 65 years of age and older continues to rise (Yorkston, Bourgeois, & Baylor, 2010).

115

Poor communication between healthcare providers and seniors is well known to be associated with worse health outcomes (Yorkston et al., 2010). The 2003 National Assessment of Adult Literacy revealed that only 3% of adults age 65 and older were proficient in health literacy skills (Kutner, Greenberg, Jin, & Paulsen, 2006). For senior patients, these factors can reduce adherence to and persistence with medication regimens (Williams, Davis, Parker, & Weiss, 2002). Medication nonadherence among older adults is associated with 10% of hospital admissions, 25% of nursing home admissions, and approximately 20% of preventable adverse drug events in the community setting (Krueger, Felkey, & Berger, 2003). Communicating with older adults requires a unique understanding of patient perspectives, needs, and expectations.

Good communication entails more than simply overcoming physical limitations that may be present, such as hearing or visual impairment. Certainly, physical impairments and cognitive issues may exist, making communication with older adults more challenging. However, having the ability to listen to patient concerns and understand unique needs will help the pharmacist (or any other healthcare professional) develop a relationship based on mutual trust and understanding and allow both parties to achieve the desired goals from the interaction.

STEREOTYPES RELATED TO AGING

Communication between older adults and healthcare professionals can be hindered by stereotypes or misguided beliefs from either party. Healthcare professionals may assume that all older adults are hard of hearing and cognitively impaired. In other circumstances, hearing impairment may be mistaken for cognitive impairment or dementia. As a result, healthcare providers are often accused of communicating in a condescending manner toward older adults, speaking in an angry tone to compensate for hearing issues, and providing less critical information due to concerns about the person's ability to comprehend and remember information. Some of these stereotypes are perpetuated by the fact that normal aging does affect hearing (presbycusis), vision (presbyopia), language comprehension, and memory. It is important for healthcare providers to be aware of the inclination to stereotype when interacting with older adults. In addition, the pharmacist must take the time to listen to the patient, which is the only way to better evaluate the individual's true abilities and adjust communication to fit the situation.

Similarly, older patients often minimize medical problems or fail to report medical issues to healthcare providers. Morgan, Pendleton, Clague, and Horan (1997) surveyed 100 seniors to understand their perceptions of the significance of symptoms. They found that seniors would consider certain symptoms as a normal consequence of aging and therefore would not seek advice from a healthcare professional. In addition, if prior symptoms or complaints were minimized or shrugged off by a provider as normal or due to old age, patients may be less likely to discuss the symptoms they may be experiencing.

COMMUNICATING WITH COGNITIVELY IMPAIRED INDIVIDUALS

Cognitive changes do occur as part of normal aging, but the usual decline in mental capacity that accompanies aging does not produce changes that are severe enough to affect routine daily functioning. In more severe instances, patients with dementia (such as Alzheimer's disease) do experience cognitive changes that have an influence on their ability to work or perform routine daily functions. Patients with significant cognitive impairment or dementia most often will have a spouse, child, or caregiver involved in a medical encounter. In the latter circumstance, it is important to still include the patient in communication encounters and discussions rather than focusing the conversation only toward the spouse or caregiver. In addition, the tone (relaxed and patient but not condescending), pace of communication (avoid significant slowing of speech), and types of questions asked (simple and straightforward, without testing) are all important to consider when interacting with patients diagnosed with dementia.

CREATING AN ENVIRONMENT FOR EFFECTIVE COMMUNICATION

There are numerous strategies for creating an effective environment for communicating with older adults. Not all recommendations are applicable in every situation; the older adult population is as diverse, if not more so, as younger populations. Having the ability to assess the patient and the situation to create a thoughtful communication strategy is key to an effective interaction. The manner in which you give information is often as important as, if not more important than, the information you provide. **Table 10-1** presents several tips for communicating with older patients developed by Robinson, White, and Houchins (2006), including what to do and to avoid both verbally and nonverbally.

Table 10-1: Tips on Communicating with Older Patients	
Tip	**Reasoning**
Face patients when you speak to them, with your face at the same level.	This creates an environment suitable for exchanging conversation and allows patients with hearing impairment the opportunity to read lips.
Avoid areas with significant background noise.	Age-related hearing loss can make it more challenging for patients to understand and comprehend what is said in a setting with competing noise.

(continues)

Table 10-1: Tips on Communicating with Older Patients (Continued)

Tip	Reasoning
Begin the conversation with casual topics and familiar subjects (family, sports, weather).	This helps create a comfortable situation and sets the stage for an open exchange of information. It also lets the patient know that the healthcare professional is interested in the patient as a person and what he or she has to say.
Avoid quick shifts from topic to topic.	This prevents a reduction in comprehension; quick shifts in topics may increase confusion and make patients feel rushed and unheard.
Keep sentences and questions short and use concrete language (avoid overuse of medical jargon), which helps create a tangible image: "You should take this medication with breakfast, lunch, and dinner" rather than "You should adhere to you medications as your doctor has prescribed."	This improves comprehension and is helpful for avoiding information overload.
Do not rush the communication encounter.	This calms any fears and anxieties that patients may have about medical issues and their own aging and provides an environment of mutual respect for each person's time.
Actively listen: Look at patients when they are speaking to you and acknowledge what they are saying with nonverbal gestures, such as nodding, or verbally, by repeating back what is stated, so that the patient knows you have heard what has been said.	Patients often do not feel listened to. This practice helps the patient feel valued and that what they have to say is important.
Ask about the patient's own wishes, goals, and preferences.	This assists the healthcare professional in evaluating what the patient's priorities are, which will help guide decision making.
Provide choices to ease decision making.	This incorporates patient desires and priorities, builds trust, enhances satisfaction and treatment adherence, and improves health outcomes.

LEARN, PRACTICE, AND ASSESS ● ▲ ■
CASE STUDY EXERCISES

● **LEARN:** Example Patient Dialogues

Directions: Read the following case study. After completing Patient Dialogue One and Patient Dialogue Two, consider the differences between them and answer the questions provided.

PATIENT CASE

Bill Jones is a 76-year-old male patient who was seen in the emergency room 4 days ago for new-onset atrial fibrillation. He presented with palpitations (rapid heart rate) and was admitted to the hospital overnight. He was started on metoprolol XL 50 mg daily and warfarin 5 mg daily. The patient is referred to the pharmacist-managed anticoagulation clinic for follow up of warfarin management. He is in the clinic today with his wife to see the pharmacist for the first time.

PATIENT DIALOGUE ONE

Pharmacist: Hello, Mr. Jones. I am the pharmacist you are to see today.

Patient's wife: Hi. Bill does not hear very well.

Pharmacist: Okay, that is not a problem. We will figure it all out. (*Speaking to the wife but looking at the computer.*) It looks like your husband was seen in the emergency room for AFib. Is this a new problem for him?

Patient's wife: Uh, well, I am not sure what AFib is. They told him he had a heart rhythm problem and started him on some new medications. They told us we needed to see the pharmacist, but I am not clear why.

Pharmacist: (*Speaking to the wife.*) AFib is an arrhythmia that is pretty common among older adults. It's my job to adjust the dose of the warfarin medication he was started on.

Patient's wife: We had some questions about the warfarin. Bill's brother was on warfarin before, and he had some serious bleeding. We are concerned that the same kind of thing can happen to Bill.

Pharmacist: (*Speaking to the wife.*) Warfarin can increase the risk of bleeding, but it is a useful medication for AFib, and this is what Dr. Smith prescribed for him. It is very important that he take the medication every day. Also, there are a lot of drug interactions with warfarin as well as dietary factors that can interact with warfarin therapy. We will need to talk about those. But, first, let's check his INR and see where we are at. (*The pharmacist starts prepping the patient's finger for point-of-care testing of the INR.*)

Patient: (*To his wife.*) What is he saying? I didn't catch much of it.

Pharmacist: (*To Mr. Jones, in a loud voice.*) It is okay, Mr. Jones. We are going to get you all squared away after we stick your finger. (*The patient shakes his head at his wife and they remain silent for the remainder of the appointment, tuning out what the pharmacist is saying.*)

PATIENT DIALOGUE TWO

Pharmacist: Hello, Mr. Jones. I am Mike, the pharmacist you are to see today.

Patient's wife: Hi. Bill does not hear very well.

Pharmacist: (*To the wife.*) Okay. Is your husband able to read lips?

Patient's wife: He can understand pretty well if you look directly at him and speak a little slower.

Pharmacist: (*Looking at Mr. Jones and speaking at a slower pace*). I am going to have you sit here so that I can look at you both. Mr. Jones, tell me what brings you to the clinic today.

Patient: I had some problems with my heart and had to go to the emergency room. I was started on a couple of new medications, and they told me to come in to see the pharmacist today. I am not sure why I am seeing the pharmacist rather than my doctor

Pharmacist: I will do my best to answer your questions. I work closely with your doctor to evaluate medications, like warfarin, which is one of your new medications. Tell me what you know about warfarin.

Patient: Well, I know some people call it rat poison. My brother used to take it, and he had some serious bleeding with it. I am a little worried that will happen to me.

Pharmacist: I can understand why the bleeding is a worry for you. Warfarin is a blood thinner. That is one of the reasons you were asked to see me today. My job is to closely monitor how thin your blood is while you are taking this medicine. What were you told about warfarin?

Patient: Not much, just that I needed to take it every day, and that I would need to have blood tests to check my levels.

Pharmacist: That is correct. Warfarin is often used for heart rhythm problems. The rhythm you have is called atrial fibrillation, or an irregular heartbeat. When this happens, you are at higher risk of having a stroke. Warfarin reduces your risk of having a stroke.

Patient: How often do I have to have blood tests? I hate having blood drawn.

Pharmacist: We may have to see you for blood tests every 5 to 7 days at first, but once we have your dose at the right level, we can stretch it out to 4 weeks between testing. I have a machine that allows us to just prick your finger for blood tests. How does that sound?

Patient: Yes, that makes me feel a little better.

Pharmacist: Okay, great. We have to work together to get your blood level where it needs to be. Let's discuss the signs and symptoms of bleeding so that you can know what to look out for so that you don't have the serious problem your brother had.

Discussion Questions for the **LEARN** Exercise

1. Compare and discuss how the pharmacist interacted with the patient(s) in the two dialogues. Which verbal and nonverbal communication strategies did the pharmacist in Dialogue Two use to help the patient understand the conversation?
2. Consider how the pharmacist in Dialogue One approached the patient. Unfortunately, this is how many healthcare professionals treat older patients. Discuss which stereotypes this pharmacist's behavior represents.
3. This text discusses tips for communicating with older patients. Which ones were applied in Dialogue Two?
4. Mr. Jones has impaired hearing but shows no signs of cognitive impairment. How might the pharmacist adjust his communication if Mr. Jones were showing signs of cognitive impairment?

LEARN, PRACTICE, AND ASSESS
CASE STUDY EXERCISES

 PRACTICE: Build Your Own Dialogue

Directions: Now it is time to *practice* what you have learned about the topic of this chapter. Reflecting on concepts from this chapter and the patient dialogues in the LEARN exercise, develop your own pharmacist–patient dialogue using the following patient information and guidance questions.

PATIENT CASE

Raymond Jackson is a 78-year-old African-American male who was seen in the emergency room 4 days ago for new-onset congestive heart failure. He presented with 3+ pitting edema in legs and feet, shortness of breath, and jugular venous distention. He was admitted to the hospital overnight and was placed on furosemide 80 mg daily and Metoprolol XL 100 mg daily. The patient is referred to the ambulatory heart failure clinic for follow up of medication management. He is in the clinic today with his wife to see the pharmacist for the first time.

As you plan your dialogue, keep in mind what you have learned about communicating with older patients. Use the following questions to help plan and assess your dialogue.

1. An important part of planning a dialogue is setting goals for the conversation. Given the patient's situation, what would you like to accomplish in this dialogue? Be sure to think about both short- and long-term goals. For instance, you may want to learn what the patient knows about his recent diagnosis of congestive heart failure and make sure he understands how to take his medications, but a more important goal may be to communicate to the new patient that you want to listen to what he has to say, and would like to better understand his concerns and needs.

2. Every older patient is different and may have a variety of communication barriers that hinder their medication adherence or understanding. Discuss how you plan to uncover any physical or cognitive barriers that this patient may have to adhering to his medication regimen. Also, how might you address them in your conversation?

3. It is important to plan both the verbal and nonverbal strategies you will use with older patients. What type of tone do you plan to take when talking to the patient? What pace will you plan for, and where will you have this conversation? What types of questions do you plan to ask the patient?

4. As you plan your dialogue, review the tips for communicating with older adults in this chapter. Which tips do you plan to incorporate into your dialogue?

5. How do you plan to communicate and engage the patient's wife? It is important to inquire of the patient's desires and wishes. Therefore, it is necessary to discover the patient's desired role of his spouse in his health care. How do you plan to discover what the patient desires about his spouse's involvement in the conversation?

YOUR DIALOGUE HERE

LEARN, PRACTICE, AND ASSESS
CASE STUDY EXERCISES

ASSESS: Build Your Own Dialogue

Directions: Now it is time to *assess* what you have learned about the topic of this chapter. In this exercise, no guidance questions are provided. Reflect on what you have learned from the LEARN and PRACTICE exercises, and develop your own pharmacist–patient dialogue using the following patient information.

PATIENT CASE

An 82-year-old male widower presents to your pharmacy with his daughter to pick up his prescriptions. The patient's daughter is visiting due to the patient's recent diagnosis of dementia. You notice that today's medication refills are 12 days late. The patient lives alone.

YOUR DIALOGUE HERE

DISCUSSION QUESTIONS

1. What experiences or characteristics do you have that may prepare you for communicating with older patients?
2. Which communication strategies do you plan to utilize when working with older patients?
3. The U.S. population change trend is that more and more people will live longer while trying to manage various long-term illnesses. What should your pharmacy (or organization) and the pharmacy profession do to specifically meet the needs of this population?
4. Media often portray older people as dependent, unsociable, disengaged, or difficult. In what ways might such stereotypes affect patient–pharmacist communication?

REFERENCES

Administration on Aging, U.S. Department of Health and Human Services. (2014). *A profile of older Americans: 2014*. Retrieved from http://www.aoa.gov /Aging_Statistics/Profile/2014/docs/2014-Profile.pdf

Kutner M, Greenberg E, Jin Y, Paulsen C. (2006). *The health literacy of America's adults: results from the 2003 National Assessment of Adult*. Retrieved from http://nces .ed.gov/pubsearch/pubsinfo.asp?pubid=2006483

Krueger, K. P., Felkey, B. G., & Berger, B. A. (2003). Improving adherence and persistence: A review and assessment of interventions and description of steps toward a national adherence initiative. *Journal of the American Pharmacists Association, 43*(6), 668–679.

Morgan, R., Pendleton, N., Clague, J. E., & Horan, M. A. (1997). Older people's perceptions about symptoms. *British Journal of General Practice, 47*(420), 427–430.

Robinson, T. E., II, White, G. L., & Houchins, J. C. (2006). Improving communication with older patients: Tips from the literature. *Family Practice Management, 13*(8), 73–78.

Williams, M. V., Davis, T., Parker, R. M., & Weiss, B. D. (2002). The role of health literacy in patient-physician communication. *Family Medicine, 34*(5), 383–389.

Yorkston, K. M., Bourgeois, M. S., & Baylor, C. R. (2010). Communication and aging. *Physical Medicine and Rehabilitation Clinics of North America, 21*(2), 309–319.

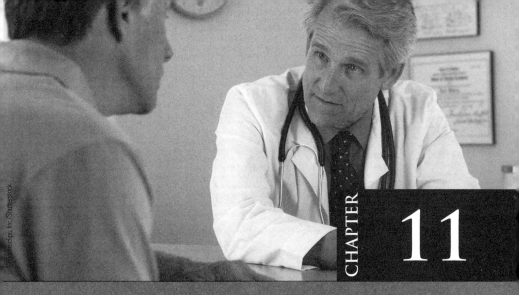

CHAPTER 11

COMMUNICATING WITH PATIENTS WITH PHYSICAL DISABILITIES

LEARNING OBJECTIVES

At the end of this chapter, students should be able to:

▸ Recognize the pharmacist's role and responsibilities in serving patients with physical disabilities.

▸ Discuss ways in which vision and hearing impairments interfere with a patient's ability to pursue healthcare needs.

▸ Identify and apply various communication tools to serve the pharmacy needs of patients with vision and hearing impairments.

KEY TERMS

Disability as contexually grounded

Legally disabled individual

Disability medical model

Social model

Under the Americans with Disabilities Act (ADA), Congress determined that an individual is **legally disabled**, and therefore deserving of legal protection against discrimination, if he or she has a physical or mental impairment that substantially limits a major life activity, has a record of such an impairment, or is regarded as having such an impairment. Patients with disabilities are a particularly important group to consider compared to nondisabled patients. They use disproportionately more healthcare services and resources but report having poorer health outcomes and being less satisfied with the quality of care received (Smith, Roth, Okoro, Kimberlin, & Odedina, 2011).

As suggested by the World Health Organization definition (n.d.), *disability* is indeed an umbrella term that captures a variety of conditions and circumstances that may limit or impair one's ability to fully participate in various activities. Consider the following disability statistics identified by the 2011 American Community Survey (Cornell University, 2013):

- The racial disparity in disability prevalence in the United States is worth noting. Native Americans and African Americans had the highest prevalence of disability among working-aged people (21–64 years): 18% and 14.2%, respectively. Asians had the lowest level of prevalence at 6.3%.
- Disability frequency also increased with age, ranging from 0.8% of persons age 4 and under, to 36.8% of persons age 65 and older, to 50.7% of persons age 75 and older.
- About 2.2% of the population reported a vision disability (defined as having difficulty seeing even when wearing glasses), and 3.4% reported a hearing disability (defined as having serious difficulty hearing).

PERSPECTIVES ON DISABILITIES

How we conceptualize disabilities may influence which solutions or interventions are generated. For instance, Smith and colleagues (2011) distinguished the medical model of disability from the social model. The **medical model** views persons with disabilities as individuals with physiological problems who need assistance or a curative solution to the problem. In contrast, the **social model** views the disability not as a problem of the individual but focuses instead on the disadvantages he or she experiences in society as a result of these disabilities. In the case of deafness, a provider functioning exclusively in the medical model will likely see the hearing impairment as a physiological deficiency that needs medical interventions (such as implants), whereas someone in the social model will likely make an effort to understand and recognize the patient's unique needs and cultural identity as a deaf person. It is important not to view these two models as mutually exclusive. One can embrace medical interventions that improve the lives of individuals with disabilities while respecting the patient's identity as shaped by his or her disability.

There is also considerable momentum in disability advocacy to move to defining **disability as contextually grounded**. (Kaplan, n.d.). In other words, rather than tying disability to certain acknowledged diagnostic categories, the movement defines disability as a contextual variable that changes over time in relation to circumstances. In this definition, disability is a product of an interaction between a person's characteristics, such as physical abilities or social characteristics, and the environment's characteristics (built or natural). This places more responsibility on healthcare providers because our ability to provide needed accommodations may make the difference between *enabling* and *disabling* patients as they seek to achieve optimum care.

COMMUNICATION NEEDS OF PATIENTS WITH DISABILITIES: MYTHS AND FACTS

Those with disabilities commonly experience difficulty navigating the insurance system, finding and obtaining approval to visit specialists, and obtaining durable medical equipment. Estimates suggest that these factors obstruct or delay care for as many as 30% to 50% of adults with disabilities (National Council on Disability, 2009). A common barrier known to affect the quality of care that people with disabilities receive is a lack of competency and awareness among healthcare providers. Patients often complain that their providers lack basic understanding of their disabilities and needs, and they find their provider's lack of willingness or inability to provide accommodations frustrating. Consider the following misperceptions versus facts regarding disabilities:

- *Myth*: Disabilities are visible.
  Fact: Disabilities, including physical disabilities, are often invisible.
- *Myth*: Deaf persons can speech read and lip read.
  Fact: Many cannot speech read, and even the best speech reader is believed to capture only about 30% of a typical conversation.
- *Myth*: American Sign Language is just English-on-hand.
  Fact: Sign language is not English and has no written equivalent in English. This means that a deaf person may have a hard time reading written materials.
- *Myth*: Individuals who are blind or visually impaired are helpless and require constant assistance.
  Fact: Individuals who are blind or visually impaired are more independent than people often give them credit for. Many individuals embrace their blindness rather than seeing it as a disability.
- *Myth*: People who are blind or visually impaired cannot read.
  Fact: Computer technologies and newly invented auxiliary devices have made nearly all print materials accessible to individuals who are blind or visually impaired.

STRATEGIES FOR ASSISTING INDIVIDUALS WITH VISUAL AND HEARING IMPAIRMENTS

Drainoni and colleagues (2006) reviewed various barriers that cause individuals with disabilities to experience more challenges and poorer outcomes in healthcare settings and classified them into three categories: *structural, financial,* and *personal/cultural.* While individual pharmacies and pharmacy professionals cannot do much to alleviate financial barriers for patients, they can improve their patients' experience by recognizing and addressing structural and personal/cultural barriers.

Structural barriers, such as transportation challenges or space limitations, make it difficult for patients to navigate and interact with the physical environment. A *New York Times* article shared strategies that pharmacy chains like Walgreens are utilizing to better connect pharmacists with their patients at a personal level, including redesigning its consultation area to better facilitate conversations (Japsen, 2011). See **Figure 11-1** for a photo of such a consultation area in a pharmacy. Consider the pharmacy settings with which you are familiar. How difficult would it be for someone who is wheelchair-bound to navigate the environment and interact with the pharmacist? What about other forms of disabilities?

Some strategies that may help reduce structural barriers in a pharmacy setting include making your facility, especially the consultation area,

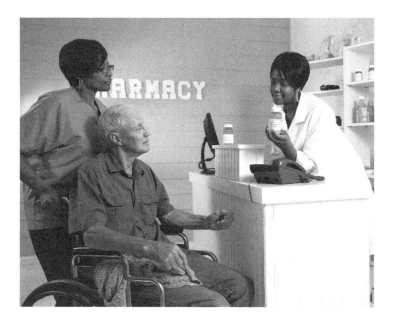

Figure 11-1   A community pharmacy consultation area
©FStop123/Getty Images

wheelchair accessible. Under the ADA Standards for Accessible Design, an accessible doorway must have a minimum clear opening width of 32" when the door is opened to 90°, with a minimum aisle width of 36". See the United States Access Board (2010) for more information regarding requirements that apply to various healthcare organizations.

Another strategy is to *make communication accessible* to individuals with hearing- and vision-related disabilities. This may include printed materials, prescription labels, and consultation with a pharmacist. For instance, a collaborative project between the American Society of Consultant Pharmacists Foundation and the American Foundation for the Blind produced a set of guidelines on how to make prescription labels and medication information accessible for those with vision loss (American Society of Consultant Pharmacists Foundation, 2008). For hearing-impaired patients, auxiliary aids and services must be offered to ensure effective communication, which is a legal obligation of all healthcare providers under the ADA. The National Association of the Deaf (n.d.) provides more information regarding healthcare providers' obligations to provide communication accommodations.

In addition, it helps to *display signage* to welcome individuals with disabilities. Consider printing a welcome sign in sign language, or posting a simple message encouraging patients to discuss with you any specific needs for accommodations. Such gestures may be particularly useful for individuals with less visible disabilities or for those who are uncomfortable discussing their needs with strangers.

Personal/cultural barriers refer to difficulties patients experience as a result of pharmacy professionals showing insensitivity or lack of respect while serving them. These may be unconsciously done; the pharmacist may not intend to be disrespectful but will still appear insensitive due to a lack of awareness or experience. Here are some general strategies to consider for this category of barriers:

- Educate yourself and other staff members to increase awareness of and knowledge about disabilities and patient needs. This may include continuous education opportunities via online or face-to-face sources sponsored by various community organizations. Community advocacy organizations are useful resources that often offer workshops to raise awareness about various disabilities.
- Be mindful of every patient's unique identity and right to optimum care, whether they are able-bodied or not. Know that disease and disability are related but different. To best assist a patient, it is important to know which diagnosis the patient has and, more important, what the patient perceives of the diagnosis, how the disease affects his or her daily routines, and the patient's health goals.
- When in doubt, ask the patient. All disabilities are not equal. A simple yet effective strategy is to ask the patient about his or her needs and which accommodations, if any, are necessary.

LEARN, PRACTICE, AND ASSESS
CASE STUDY EXERCISES

● LEARN: Example Patient Dialogues

Directions: Read the following case study. After completing Patient Dialogue One and Patient Dialogue Two, consider the differences between them and answer the questions provided.

PATIENT CASE

Phillip Smith is a 48-year-old male who has been legally blind since the age of 3. He lives by himself and is very functional. He uses a cane to guide him when walking in familiar places and a guide dog when in unfamiliar locations. Mr. Smith's locally owned independent pharmacy, which he had been using for the past 20 years, recently closed, and he is trying a new chain pharmacy near his home. He had his prescriptions transferred to the new pharmacy and arrives to pick them up for the first time.

PATIENT DIALOGUE ONE

Pharmacist: Hello, sir. (*Notices the guide dog and is startled.*) Oh, um, animals are not allowed in the store, sir! (*Frowns.*)

Patient: Ma'am, this is my guide dog. I am blind.

Pharmacist: Oh, I AM SO SORRY (*starts talking louder*). WE HAVE NEVER HAD A BLIND CUSTOMER BEFORE. SHOULD I COME OUT TO HELP YOU?

Patient: No, I am fine (*with frustration*). I just need to pick up my prescriptions that were transferred from Home Pharmacy down the street that just closed.

Pharmacist: Okay, let me get your name and I can quickly see if your prescriptions are ready so that you can get this thing—oh, I mean dog—out of here. You can have a seat so you don't have to stand for so long.

Patient: I AM FINE RIGHT HERE!

(The pharmacist finds the prescriptions and provides them to the patient.)

Pharmacist: Do you have any questions?

Patient: No, I have been taking these pills for years. This is my first time at this pharmacy and I guarantee you it will be my last! (*The patient walks off led by his guide dog.*)

PATIENT DIALOGUE TWO

Pharmacist: Hello, sir. (*Notices the guide dog and is startled.*) Oh, um, animals are not allowed in the store, sir!

Patient: Ma'am, this is my guide dog. I am blind.

Pharmacist: Oh, sir, I am so sorry, please forgive me. Welcome to our pharmacy. How can I help you?

Patient: Oh, it's okay. I am here to pick up my prescriptions that were transferred here from Home Pharmacy down the street that just closed.

Pharmacist: Sure, I can help you with that. I am glad that you chose us to provide your medication needs. We will do all we can to ensure that you made the right choice.

Patient: That's great. I feel pretty good about the decision already.

(The pharmacist locates the prescriptions and provides them to the patient.)

Pharmacist: Do you have any questions about your medications, sir?

Patient: No, I don't. I have been taking these pills for almost 20 years now. I appreciate your asking.

Pharmacist: Sir, I would really like to know more about your disability to learn more about you and how I can better serve you.

Patient: Wow, I have never had anyone ask me that. I have been legally blind since I was 3 years old. I have learned to be functional with minimal help from others. The pharmacy that I used to use provided me with braille prescription bottles and braille patient information. Is that something you offer?

Pharmacist: Oh, this is good information (*takes notes of what patient stated*). I will certainly check to see if we can provide braille prescription bottles and patient information. Is there anything else we can do to better serve you? We are so glad that you have chosen our pharmacy and we want to make your pharmacy transition as seamless as possible.

Patient: Thank you so much. It would be great if you could provide my dog Lucy treats when we come in (*smiles*)—just kidding!

Pharmacist: (*Laughs.*) Oh, I was adding that to my list (*smiles*). Please let us know if there is ever anything we can do better to meet your needs and provide the best possible service to you. Thank you again, and I look forward to seeing you back here soon. It was very nice meeting you.

Patient: I will be back! Thanks for your interest in learning more about my needs and how to meet them. I really appreciate your service.

Discussion Questions for the **LEARN** Exercise

1. What communication errors were made in Dialogue One to possibly offend the patient?
2. Consider the pharmacist's verbal communication in Dialogue Two. What did he or she do differently to win the respect and trust of this new patient?
3. This text discusses some myths about people with disabilities. What, if any, are illustrated in Dialogue One?
4. This chapter discusses the structural, financial, and personal/cultural barriers that individuals with disabilities may face while seeking care. Which specific barriers might someone like the patient in this example face when seeking care? How might the pharmacist help address these barriers?

LEARN, PRACTICE, AND ASSESS
CASE STUDY EXERCISES

▲ PRACTICE: Build Your Own Dialogue

Directions: Now it is time to *practice* what you have learned about the topic of this chapter. Reflecting on concepts from this chapter and the patient dialogues in the LEARN exercise, develop your own pharmacist–patient dialogue using the following patient information and guidance questions.

PATIENT CASE

Jodi Dillon is a single 44-year-old female who has been hearing impaired since she was an infant. She is being discharged from the hospital after having her first heart attack while mowing her lawn. She has a history of high blood pressure and was on Micardis HCT 40/12.5 mg daily. She did not monitor her blood pressure at home and did not follow up with her physician due to feelings of discomfort and mistreatment by her physician. The cardiology clinical pharmacist is consulted to provide medication discharge counseling for Ms. Dillon regarding her new medications (including how to take them): Metoprolol 50 mg BID, Lisinopril 40 mg daily, Atorvastatin 10 mg daily, and aspirin 81 mg daily. Due to her previous physician interactions, she appears apprehensive during your initial consultation. A sign language interpreter is present during the interaction.

As you plan your dialogue, keep in mind what you have learned about communicating to patients with disabilities. Use the following questions to help plan and assess your dialogue.

1. An important part of planning a dialogue is setting goals for the conversation. Given the patient's situation, what would you like to accomplish in this dialogue? Be sure to think about both short-term long-term goals. For instance, you may want to immediately understand her disability, address her apprehension, and make sure she understands how to take her medicines. At the same time, a long-term goal may be to build rapport with her and earn her trust in you as a competent and caring healthcare provider.

2. The patient's feelings of discomfort and distrust toward her physician exist as a potential barrier to your communication with her. How might this affect your dialogue with the patient? How will you overcome this barrier?

3. How will you ensure the patient's understanding of the education you are providing about her medications?

4. How will you communicate to the patient through the interpreter? Be sure to consider how you will use eye contact, to whom your questions will be addressed, and how you will manage the three-way flow of information.

5. It is important to ensure that the patient feels comfortable talking to you and that she understands how to take her medications. Which nonverbal cues might the patient display that she feels comfortable with you and understands your medication education?

YOUR DIALOGUE HERE

LEARN, PRACTICE, AND ASSESS
CASE STUDY EXERCISES

◻ ASSESS: Build Your Own Dialogue

Directions: Now it is time to *assess* what you have learned about the topic of this chapter. In this exercise, no guidance questions are provided. Reflect on what you have learned from the LEARN and PRACTICE exercises, and develop your own pharmacist–patient dialogue using the following patient information.

PATIENT CASE

Betty McKenzie is a 55-year-old female who is visually impaired and has to use a magnifying glass to see most printed materials. She arrives at the pharmacy to pick up her new prescription for Detrol LA 4 mg daily for overactive bladder. The patient is provided her prescription in a bag and asked if she has any questions. She says she has never taken the medication before, so the pharmacist goes over the written informational pamphlet and instructs the patient to read it. The pharmacist is unaware of the patient's physical disability.

YOUR DIALOGUE HERE

DISCUSSION QUESTIONS

1. Can you find any training guide or manual for pharmacy staff regarding how to provide care for and interact with customers and patients with disabilities, such as those who are visually or hearing impaired?
2. Which tools are available in community pharmacies to improve communication with visually and hearing-impaired patients?
3. As discussed in this text, there are structural, financial, and personal/ cultural barriers that must be addressed in order to improve the healthcare experience for disabled individuals. Which barriers do you think pharmacists ought to pay more attention to when serving these patients?
4. Consider media portrayals of individuals who have various forms of disabilities. Some have argued that they tend to be portrayed unfairly and in a negative light. How might such media portrayals affect the healthcare experience of individuals with disabilities?

REFERENCES

American Society of Consultant Pharmacists Foundation. (2008). *Guidelines for prescription labeling and consumer medication information for people with vision loss.* Retrieved from http://www.ascpfoundation.org/downloads/Rx-CMI%20 Guidelines%20vision%20loss-FINAL2.pdf

Cornell University. (2013). *Disability statistics.* Retrieved from http:// disabilitystatistics.org

Drainoni, M-L., Lee-Hood, E., Tobias, C., Bachman, S. S., Andrew, J., & Maisels, L. (2006). Cross-disability experiences of barriers to health-care access. Journal of Disability Policy Studies, *17*(2), 101–115.

Japsen, B. (2011, October 21). Out from behind the counter. *The New York Times.* Retrieved from http://www.nytimes.com/2011/10/22/business /at-walgreens-pharmacists-urged-to-mix-with-public.html

Kaplan, D. (n.d.). The definition of disability. *The Center for an Accessible Society.* Retrieved from http://www.accessiblesociety.org/topics /demographics-identity/dkaplanpaper.htm

National Association of the Deaf. (n.d.). *Questions and answers for health care providers.* Retrieved from http://www.nad.org/issues/health-care/providers /questions-and-answers

National Council on Disability. (2009). *The current state of health care for people with disabilities.* Retrieved from http://www.ncd.gov/publications/2009 /Sept302009#exesum

Smith, W. T., Roth, J. J., Okoro, O., Kimberlin, C., & Odedina, F. T. (2011). Disability in cultural competency pharmacy education. *American Journal of Pharmaceutical Education, 75*(2), 26.

Steinberg, A. G., Barnett, S., Meador, H. E., Wiggins, E. A., & Zazove, P. (2006). Health care system accessibility: Experiences and perceptions of deaf people. *Journal of General Internal Medicine, 21*(3), 260–266.

United States Access Board. (2010). *ADA standards.* Retrieved from http://www.access-board.gov/guidelines-and-standards/buildings-and-sites/about-the-ada-standards/ada-standards

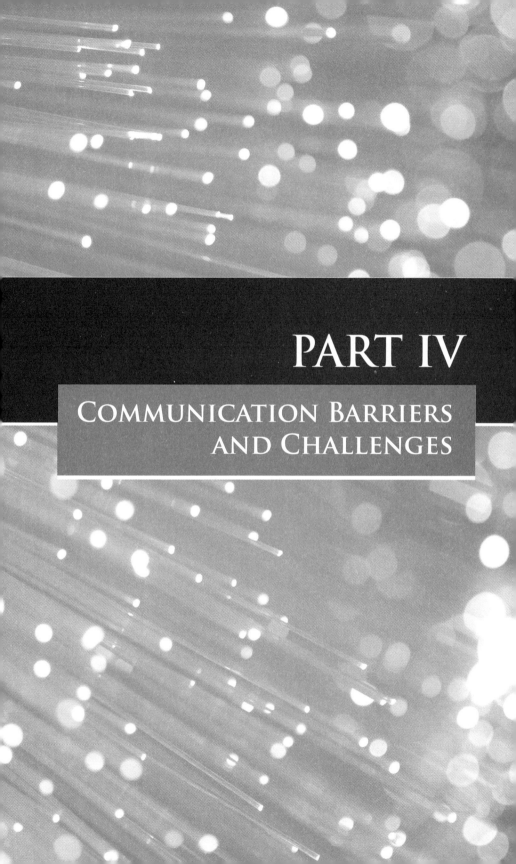

PART IV

COMMUNICATION BARRIERS AND CHALLENGES

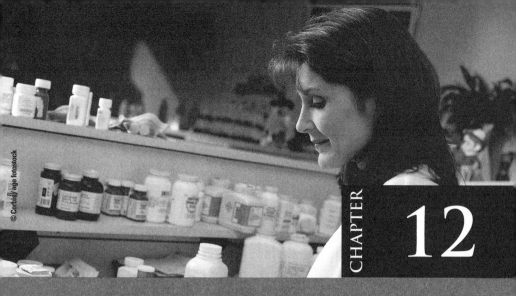

12

ENVIRONMENTAL AND PSYCHOLOGICAL BARRIERS TO COMMUNICATION

LEARNING OBJECTIVES

At the end of this chapter, students should be able to:

▸ Recognize various types of barriers that may affect pharmacist–patient communication.

▸ Identify strategies to address environmental and psychological communication barriers.

▸ Identify specific behaviors of ineffective listening.

▸ Discuss communication strategies to assess communication barriers and improve communication quality.

KEY TERMS

Defensive listening or aggressive listening

Environmental barriers

Noise

Perception-checking

Pseudo-listening

Psychological barriers

Selective listening

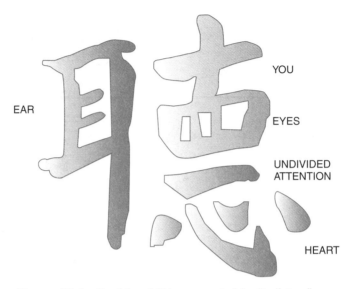

EAR

YOU

EYES

UNDIVIDED
ATTENTION

HEART

Figure 12-1 Traditional Chinese symbol for "to listen."

Communication does not occur in a vacuum. In a pharmacist's daily conversations with patients, colleagues, or other healthcare professionals, there are a multitude of factors, both internal and external, that may influence how people interpret and respond to what is communicated in the process. This is referred to as *noise* in the transactional model of communication. **Noise** is anything that interferes with the encoding and decoding of a message. In other words, these are barriers that may prevent you or the other person from paying attention to something important being said, or cause the parties to misunderstand one another. If not addressed, barriers can cause a communication breakdown between conversation partners.

Many of us take communication for granted. Think about listening, for instance. People often mistakenly believe that, because they have been listening all of their lives, they must be good at it. We must be cognizant of how various communication barriers can limit our ability to listen effectively. Look at the traditional Chinese symbol for the verb "to listen," shown in **Figure 12-1**. The left side represents the ear, and the right side includes the symbol for the eyes as well as the symbol for "one heart," which also means "undivided attention." In other words, listening involves not only our ears but also our eyes, and to be effective listeners our attention must not be divided. It is easy to see why so many of us fail at the art of listening.

TYPES OF COMMUNICATION BARRIERS

In a recent systematic literature review of pharmacist and consumer perceptions, several barriers were identified as limiting a pharmacist's ability to promote patient and community health, including lack of training, privacy concerns, and time limitations (Eades, Ferguson, & O'Carroll, 2011). Some barriers may affect certain populations more than others. For example, Cleland and colleagues (2012) interviewed community pharmacists who serve non-English-speaking immigrants and identified such key barriers as communication challenges, privacy concerns when family and friends are used as interpreters, and frustration with the consultation process.

Consider the different types of barriers that may influence the typical pharmacist–patient communication. The major types of barriers are environmental barriers and psychological barriers.

Environmental barriers, also known as *external noise*, refer to anything in the physical or social background that makes effective communication difficult, such as other conversations taking place, a poor connection with phone conversations, or a lack of privacy for discussing personal information.

Psychological barriers, also known as *internal noise*, include personal biases, perceptions, or other cognitive processes that interfere with our ability to effectively listen and contribute to a conversation. While environmental barriers often make the sending and receiving of communication signals difficult, psychological barriers are more likely to lead to misinterpretation, communication breakdowns, or even conflicts. Environmental barriers are often visible to the communicators involved; psychological barriers may influence our ability to communicate, even though we may not fully realize it. As communicators, the key is to always be aware of which barriers may exist in the environment and in the minds of the people involved.

Consider the following list of possible barriers and how each may influence communication between the pharmacist and the patient:

- After receiving news of extended work hours, the pharmacist is in a bad mood when the patient approaches him.
- The patient believes that his previous pharmacist was rude and disrespectful and decided to switch to another pharmacy. As he approaches the pharmacist, he wonders how the experience will turn out.
- The patient wants to ask the pharmacist about the side effects of a medication she has been on for a few months. She has been having more depressive thoughts since being on it and wonders if it is a side effect of the medication. However, there is a line waiting behind her and there is not a private patient consultation area.
- As the pharmacist greets the patient and processes the prescription, she is thinking to herself about the list of things she needs to get done before the evening rush comes in, including several phone calls she has been dreading.

As you can see, barriers are always present in our communication. Another way to think about barriers is to consider which ones are *within our control* and which ones are *beyond our control*. For instance, you may not be able to control the surrounding conversations in the background that make it harder to hear, but you can point out the need to speak a bit louder or stand closer so that you can hear one another clearly. You cannot control the patient's biases or preconceived notions that could cause him or her to misinterpret what you are saying, but you can increase the clarity of your message. To avoid misunderstanding the patient, **perception-checking** is a useful technique. To implement it, share your observation and perception of what is happening, describe what you consider to be the probable interpretations, and ask the patient for clarification to avoid misunderstanding (Coleman, 2005).

HOW TO ADDRESS COMMUNICATION BARRIERS

Communication barriers are always present and constantly changing. As a result, there is no easy way to eliminate them from our communication. Instead, we must be mindful of the barriers that are present and how they may be influencing the quality of communication. To address these barriers, we can implement the following specific actions in our daily practices:

- *Advocate for systematic changes* to remove environmental barriers. For instance, if you have observed that your patients often need or want more privacy, become an advocate for your patients by helping to create a private patient counseling area.
- *Be mindful* of your own psychological barriers. If you find yourself mentally distracted by something unrelated to the patient, remind yourself that the patient deserves your full attention. Try to shut off all internal noise prior to entering the interaction and concentrate on each patient with whom you come into contact.
- *Check perceptions.* Communication barriers are problematic because they lead to misinterpretations and miscommunication. To ensure communication accuracy, use different tools to check perceptions. To confirm that the patient has understood medication instructions, for instance, you can use the teach-back method (see the chapter on Communicating with Patients with Low Health Literacy). To ensure that you have understood the patient, you can paraphrase what you heard and ask the patient if your interpretation is correct.

PRACTICE THE ART OF ACTIVE LISTENING

In our daily lives, we mostly use four acts of communication: speaking, writing, reading, and listening. While communication barriers could influence all four, the one that is most likely to be affected is probably listening. Environmental barriers could limit our ability to hear one another clearly. Psychological barriers could lead to various types of ineffective listening (McCornack, 2009). For instance, we may be rushed or distracted in a conversation and engage in **selective listening**, which is listening to only parts of a conversation, usually the parts that interest us most. Or we may engage in **pseudo-listening**, or pretending to listen, when we know that we should be listening but feel we are unable to or simply cannot concentrate on the conversation. Psychological barriers could also lead to **defensive listening** or **aggressive listening**, which is interpreting an innocent comment as a personal attack or criticism and becoming defensive in the conversation. Our biases, prejudices, and other cognitive processes, such as feelings of insecurity or previous negative experiences, often cause defensive listening. To practice the art of active listening, the key is to silence the internal noise that may cause us to engage in these ineffective listening behaviors.

LEARN, PRACTICE, AND ASSESS
CASE STUDY EXERCISES

● **LEARN: Example Patient Dialogues**

Directions: Read the following case study. After completing Patient Dialogue One and Patient Dialogue Two, consider the differences between them and answer the questions provided.

PATIENT CASE

A 23-year-old college student had unprotected sex 2 days ago and is scared that she may be pregnant. She has a fear of doctors and healthcare professionals in general because she had a bad experience as a teenager when her male doctor called her fat and told her she "needs to stop eating like a pig." This statement caused her to begin experiencing depression symptoms such as frequent crying when looking in the mirror and limited desire to be around others. She goes to the university health services to request a prescription for emergency contraception. The prescription was called in to her local pharmacy and she arrives to pick it up, having no knowledge of how to take the medication. She arrives at 4:45 on a Monday evening during the pharmacy's busy rush hour. The pharmacist has felt stressed today due to a high prescription volume and the calling off of her second shift pharmacist due to illness. She is in the midst of a phone call with her district manager who is trying to locate a relief pharmacist to come in by 6:00 p.m. to allow the pharmacist to leave. The pharmacist has not had a break since coming in at 9:00 a.m. and she is frustrated.

PATIENT DIALOGUE ONE

Pharmacist tech: (*Approaches the patient at the counter while typing in a prescription at a computer near the counter.*) Hi, can I help you? (*Sounding rushed.*)

Patient: (*Avoiding eye contact and appearing nervous.*) Hi. I need to pick up my prescription.

Pharmacy tech: What's your name?

Patient: Courtney Long. (*Soft tone.*)

Pharmacy tech: I can't hear you, what did you say?

Patient: Courtney Long! (*Projects her voice.*)

(The technician checks the prescription bins, finds the patient's prescription bag, and returns to the patient at the counter.)

Pharmacy tech: Can you please verify your address?

Patient: 321 Piper—

Pharmacy tech: (*Cuts off the patient.*) Okay! Do you have any questions for the pharmacist?

Patient: Yes, can I speak with the pharmacist in private? (*Soft tone.*)

Pharmacy tech: (*Yelling to the pharmacist.*) Linda, this patient wants to talk to you about her prescription. (*Talking to the patient.*) Go over to the consultation window and she will be right with you.

Pharmacist: (*Takes a deep breath, turns around to look at the patient briefly while holding the phone up to ear.*) Yes, can I help you? (*Seeming rushed.*)

Patient: Never mind, it looks like you are busy. Have a nice day.

Pharmacist: You too. (*Gets back to the conversation on the phone.*)

PATIENT DIALOGUE TWO

Pharmacy tech: (*Approaches the patient at the counter while typing in a prescription at a computer near the counter.*) Hi, can I help you? (*Sounding rushed.*)

Patient: (*Avoiding eye contact and appearing nervous.*) Hi. I need to pick up my prescription.

Pharmacy tech: What's your name?

Patient: Courtney Long. (*Soft tone.*)

Pharmacy tech: I can't hear you, what did you say?

Patient: Courtney Long! (*Projects voice.*)

(The technician checks the prescription bins, finds the patient's prescription bag, and returns to the patient at the counter.)

Pharmacy tech: (*Noticing that the patient appears nervous.*) Let's go over here to the consultation window so that you can discuss your prescription with the pharmacist.

Pharmacy tech: Can you please verify your address?

Patient: 321 Piper Lane.

Pharmacy tech: Okay, great. The pharmacist will be with you shortly.

(The technician walks over to the pharmacist and tells her that she has a customer waiting to speak with her and that she seems nervous. The technician offers to get on the phone with the district manager while the pharmacist talks with the patient. The pharmacist takes a few deep breaths to relieve some frustration and reminds herself not to display any frustration to the patient.)

Pharmacist: Hi, ma'am, sorry for your wait. How can I help you?

Patient: I have this new prescription that I have never taken before. Can you tell me how to take it? (*Handing the prescription bag to the pharmacist.*)

Pharmacist: (*Looking at the label.*) Sure, I am so glad you came over to talk with me because it is very important that you take this medication as prescribed.

(The pharmacist goes on to discuss how the first pill should be taken immediately and then the next pill 12 hours later and also explains the possible side effects and when she should expect her next menstrual cycle.)

Patient: Thank you so much for taking the time to talk with me. You don't know how much this means to me!

Pharmacist: It is my pleasure. Please don't hesitate to call or stop back if you have any questions.

Discussion Questions for the **LEARN** Exercise

1. Consider the patient case and the two dialogues. Which psychological and/or environmental barriers may be affecting the patient's ability to fully engage in the conversation?
2. Which psychological and/or environmental barriers may be affecting the pharmacy professionals' ability to engage in the conversation?
3. Consider Dialogue Two. How did the pharmacy technician and pharmacist address the communication barriers with the patient? Did they use active listening? Explain why.
4. Which verbal and nonverbal strategies did the pharmacy professionals in Dialogue Two use to indicate that they genuinely wanted to listen to the patient?

LEARN, PRACTICE, AND ASSESS
CASE STUDY EXERCISES

 PRACTICE: Build Your Own Dialogue

Directions: Now it is time to *practice* what you have learned about the topic of this chapter. Reflecting on concepts from this chapter and the patient dialogues in the LEARN exercise, develop your own pharmacist–patient dialogue using the following patient information and guidance questions.

PATIENT CASE

Martin Berry, a 48-year-old Caucasian male, presents to the clinic for a medication management referral appointment with the clinical pharmacist. His past medical history is significant for hypertension and type 2 diabetes. He has previously taken the following antihypertensive medications and developed significant side effects:

- Lisinopril 20 mg daily: developed angioedema, medication was discontinued
- Hydrochlorothiazide 25 mg daily: developed gout due to increased uric acid levels
- Spironolactone 25 mg BID: developed gynecomastia

He is currently taking Amlodipine 10 mg daily and his blood pressure today is 164/108, when at his previous visit it was 150/98. His physician would like help choosing another antihypertensive to add on. The patient is very apprehensive about starting a new medication due to his significant history of developing major side effects from previous medications.

As you plan your dialogue, keep in mind what you have learned about communicating with patients in the presence of environmental and psychological barriers. Use the following questions to help plan and assess your dialogue.

1. An important part of planning a dialogue is setting goals for the conversation. Given the patient's situation, what would you like to accomplish in this dialogue? Be sure to think about both short- and long-term goals. For instance, you may want to understand and address the patient's apprehension and discuss and educate the patient on medication side effects and the importance of getting his blood pressure under control. However, a more important goal may be to reassure the patient that you want to listen to what he has to say and discuss any concerns he may have in the future.

2. In order to mentally remove communication barriers, you must first be aware of them. As you read this patient case and envision yourself as

the pharmacist, which psychological barriers do you have or may have that could interfere with your ability to effectively communicate with the patient?

3. Which barriers may the patient have that would interfere with your communication effort? How do you plan to overcome all of the barriers present?

4. As healthcare providers, we can serve as examples for our patients. The art of active listening is no different. How can you model active listening to your patient despite the presence of environmental and/or psychological barriers?

5. How will you ensure that the patient understands his new antihypertensive medication regimen and the reason for the new recommendation?

YOUR DIALOGUE HERE

LEARN, PRACTICE, AND ASSESS
CASE STUDY EXERCISES

ASSESS: Build Your Own Dialogue

Directions: Now it is time to *assess* what you have learned about the topic of this chapter. In this exercise, no guidance questions are provided. Reflect on what you have learned from the LEARN and PRACTICE exercises, and develop your own pharmacist–patient dialogue using the following patient information.

PATIENT CASE

Teresa Lang is a 42-year-old female with a history of four strokes in the past 2 years. She has been noncompliant with her medications and has been known to tell physicians what they want to hear about how she takes them. The patient has a history of depression and feels that she has nothing to live for. She presents to the primary care clinic for follow up with her physician and clinical pharmacist. The clinical pharmacist is frustrated and cannot believe she had another stroke this month.

YOUR DIALOGUE HERE

DISCUSSION QUESTIONS

1. Consider the different types of ineffective listening addressed in this chapter. Can you think of recent times when you engaged in ineffective listening? If so, which psychological barriers may have contributed to the ineffective listening?
2. Reflect on the way you listen throughout the day. Using a listening journal, document each time you listen to someone else. What are your strengths as a listener? What areas do you need to work on?
3. This text discusses several types of ineffective listening. In your listening journal, discuss the specific times you have engaged in each type. Do you observe any patterns that trigger your ineffective listening habit?
4. Some argue that, although many technologies have been developed to enhance communication, such as text messaging, they are not listener-friendly and are instead contributing to the worsening of listening skills. What is your opinion on such a belief?
5. Which techniques have been implemented in the typical community pharmacy setting to remove environmental barriers for communication? What else can be done?

REFERENCES

Cleland, J. A., Watson, M. C., Walker, L., Denison, A., Vanes, N., & Moffat, M. (2012). Community pharmacists' perceptions of barriers to communication with migrants. *International Journal of Pharmacy Practice, 20*(3), 148-154.

Coleman, M. B. (2005). *Interpersonal communication: Building your foundations for success.* Dubuque, IA: Kendall Hunt.

Eades, C. E., Ferguson, J. S., & O'Carroll, R. E. (2011). Public health in community pharmacy: A systematic review of pharmacist and consumer views. *BMC Public Health, 11*(582). doi:10.1186/1471-2458-11-582

McCornack, S. (2009). *Reflect and relate: An introduction to interpersonal communication* (2nd ed.). Boston, MA: Bedford/St. Martin's.

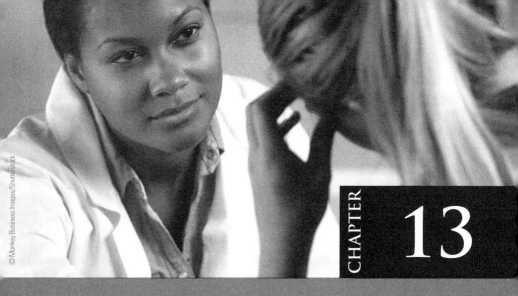

CHAPTER 13

COMMUNICATING ABOUT EMOTIONALLY CHARGED TOPICS

LEARNING OBJECTIVES

At the end of this chapter, students should be able to:

▶ Articulate the importance of conflict and conflict resolution.

▶ Recognize conflict as a multidimensional experience for both parties involved.

▶ Generate communication strategies to manage conflict.

KEY TERMS

Behavioral dimension of conflict

Cognitive dimension of conflict

Conflict

Emotional dimension of conflict

In a pharmacist's daily practice, interactions with patients, colleagues, physicians, and other members of the healthcare team offer opportunities to develop meaningful relationships. At the same time, however, conflicts may occur during such interactions. When a conversation becomes emotionally charged, conflict resolution skills are essential to preserving the relationship, be it personal or professional, while achieving communication goals.

Communication between pharmacists and patients could become emotionally charged for a variety of reasons. When patients come to a pharmacy, they may be under stress from being ill. They might be frustrated by their experience at the hospital, or at the physician's office, or in many cases with the insurance company. They may be overwhelmed and anxious to get their prescribed medications. Although the pharmacist has no control over the patient's current illness, previous experience, or how the insurance plan works, these factors will nonetheless be present in the patient encounter, and if not addressed properly, will lead to potential conflicts.

Conflicts with patients could have real implications for both the pharmacist and the patient. Unresolved conflicts make future interactions with the patient more challenging. The patient may decide not to come back to the pharmacy, which could cause an interruption in care. According to Evans, Vacca, Khanfar, and Harrington (2010), a prescription used chronically can attribute to $840 in average sales for a community pharmacy annually. The researchers estimated that losing a patient with diabetes, HIV, or chronic obstructive pulmonary disease could mean a loss of sales of well over $25,000 per year. Not only is effectively resolving conflicts with patients financially wise, it also benefits the pharmacy personnel, as conflicts have been found to significantly influence employee morale.

UNDERSTANDING CONFLICTS

Conflict is often defined as occurring between individuals with incompatible goals or needs. Although everyone has experienced conflict first hand, understanding conflict is not an easy task. Theories and models have been created to dissect and analyze conflict and ultimately to more effectively manage and resolve conflicts.

One such model states that conflicts have a cognitive dimension, an emotional dimension, and a behavioral dimension (Mayer, 2012). At the cognitive dimension, conflicts essentially reflect our beliefs about the values, needs, and goals that are incompatible with those of the other party and cause the conflict. At the emotional dimension, we have an emotional reaction to the cognitive dimension of the conflict, and the emotions might be anger, fear, bitterness, frustration, hopelessness, or helplessness. At the behavioral dimension, our behaviors and actions during the conflict are displayed, and with these actions we express our emotions and manifest our cognitive processes related to the conflict. These actions, including what we express with our words and body, could be aggressive or even violent, but they could also be constructive and collaborative. Use this model to analyze a recent conflict you were involved in and ask yourself the following questions:

- What was I *thinking* before, during, and after the conflict? What emotions did I *feel*? Which *actions* did I take to express myself in the conflict or to resolve the conflict?
- Thinking about the other party, which *actions* did the individual take to express himself or herself to resolve the conflict? What emotions did he or she *seem to be feeling*? What did he or she *seem to be thinking* before, during, and after the conflict?

Note that when observing the other party, we start by watching their actions and come to our own conclusions about the other party's emotions and thoughts. This is because behaviors are the only observable dimension of the three, and we make assumptions about one another's thoughts and feelings by observing the other person's behaviors. Keep in mind that the rule of reciprocity is relevant here, because the other person also makes assumptions about our thoughts and emotions by observing our actions. In conflict situations, it is important to be mindful of what our actions may say about our thoughts and emotions and to always bear in mind that our assumptions about the other person's thoughts and emotions may be inaccurate.

HOW TO MANAGE CONFLICTS THROUGH COMMUNICATION

- *Depersonalize the conflict situation.* At times, a patient's *actions* may lead us to see the conflict as a personal attack or a criticism of our professional skills. Such *thoughts* could lead us to *feel* defensive or hurt and as a result cause us to *behave* in a dismissive or unconstructive way. It is important to refrain from reacting to the conflict in this way, to try to keep our emotional reaction at a minimum level, and to focus on addressing the conflict and meeting the patient's needs in a professional manner.
- *Address any misunderstandings or confusion at the cognitive level.* Is the conflict caused by really incompatible goals, or could it be a result of confusion or a misunderstanding by either party? Listen to the patient to understand his or her *thoughts* about what is happening and why the patient is *feeling* frustrated or angry. For instance, the patient may not understand the complicated procedure of having a prescription filled and the steps and parties involved in the process. Or the patient may not understand how his or her insurance plan works and may blame the pharmacist for not providing the medications desired. Addressing these misunderstandings at the *cognitive* level may quickly resolve the conflict at its root.

- *Acknowledge the emotional needs of the patient.* Emotions can fuel a conflict; addressing the emotional dimension can help de-escalate it. Whether we feel the patient's emotional reaction is justified or not is irrelevant. Remember that humans do not like to be told how they should or should not feel. Instead, acknowledge the *emotions* that the patient seems to be expressing with his or her *actions* and, if appropriate, speak with empathy in a way that validates the patient's emotional needs. With this step, the patient will be more receptive to any solutions you may offer later.
- *Find a common ground with the patient.* Conflicts exist because two parties have incompatible goals or needs, or at least the two parties *think* that they do. No matter how big the gap seems between two parties, there is always a way to find and establish common ground. Providing reliable and fast service and improving the patient's health, for instance, are goals with which patients can identify. When needed, remind the patient that these are also your priorities.
- *Offer action steps that are patient-specific.* Often, patients become upset because of the things they *think* you cannot or will not do for them, such as giving them the brand-name medication they want or charging them a lower prescription copay. Instead of becoming defensive, help patients understand the things that you are willing and able to do for them; if possible, give them options to choose from as to how they want you to help them. This gives a sense of control back to the patient and may help deescalate the conflict.

Causes of conflicts for pharmacists can vary. They can be triggered by incompatible goals or needs between different individuals, teams, organizations, or even professions. The causes are often beyond the control of the pharmacist or the patient. When a communication situation involving a patient becomes emotionally charged, it is the pharmacist's responsibility to use ethical, appropriate, and effective communication strategies to resolve the conflict and maintain the relationship.

LEARN, PRACTICE, AND ASSESS
CASE STUDY EXERCISES

LEARN: Example Patient Dialogues

Directions: Read the following case study. After completing Patient Dialogue One and Patient Dialogue Two, consider the differences between them and answer the questions provided.

PATIENT CASE

A 48-year-old female who was recently hospitalized arrives at the pharmacy drive-thru window requesting to pick up her prescriptions that were sent by the hospital discharge physician. The patient went to the hospital 4 days ago due to shortness of breath, productive cough with green sputum, and chest pain. During her hospitalization, she was diagnosed with pneumonia and started on an antibiotic and mucolytic (an agent that helps to break up mucus), which were also sent to her pharmacy to continue for 10 more days at home. The patient was discharged from the hospital at 4:00 p.m. today, but her husband did not get off work until 10:00 p.m. and so could not pick her up until then. The patient is ready to get home because she hated being in the hospital and also disliked the hospital food.

PATIENT DIALOGUE ONE

Overnight pharmacist: Hello, how can I help you?

Patient's husband: We are here to pick up my wife's prescriptions that the hospital called in for her. Her name is Susan Brewer.

Pharmacist: (*The pharmacist moves to the computer to look up the prescriptions and then retrieves the bagged prescriptions from the prescription bins. She walks back to the window.*) I have two prescriptions here for you. One is for an antibiotic and another to help break up mucus in your respiratory tract. Your total is $84.50.

Patient's husband: (*Yelling.*) WHAT?! It costs that much for only two prescriptions?

Patient: (*Yelling.*) THAT IS RIDICULOUS! Did you run this through my insurance?

Pharmacist: Yes, I did. Can you come inside while I check to see the reason for the cost because there are some cars behind you?

Patient's husband: (*Yelling and frustrated.*) My wife just got out of the hospital and I just got off work. This is ridiculous how much you are charging us for just two prescriptions.

Pharmacist: I am not charging you this price. This is the price your insurance is charging. Can you please come inside?

(The patient and her husband speed off from the drive-thru window without saying anything. Two minutes later they walk up to the counter, frustrated and angry.)

Pharmacist: Ma'am, I checked into your prescriptions and it looks like this is not a preferred medication that your insurance company will pay for, and they have charged you the highest copay of $75.

Patient: I refuse to pay this. I have been in the hospital for 4 days, and I had to wait on my husband to leave and I am exhausted. I just want to get my medicine and go home! You are preventing me from getting my medicine by charging this ridiculous price. Where is your manager?

Pharmacist: (*Yelling with frustration.*) I am NOT charging you this price. Once again, THIS is the price YOUR insurance company is charging. This is not my fault and I will be glad to get the manager because you will not talk to me that way. I don't have time for this. (*Walking away.*)

(The argument escalates and the store manager comes over to calm the patient and the pharmacist.)

PATIENT DIALOGUE TWO

Overnight pharmacist: Hello, how can I help you?

Patient's husband: We are here to pick up my wife's prescriptions that the hospital called in for her. Her name is Susan Brewer.

Pharmacist: (*The pharmacist moves to the computer to look up the prescriptions and then retrieves the bagged prescriptions from the prescription bin. She walks back to window.*) I have two prescriptions here for you. One is for an antibiotic and another to help break up mucus in your respiratory tract. Your total is $84.50.

Patient's husband: (*Yelling.*) WHAT?! It costs that much for only two prescriptions?

Patient: (*Yelling.*) THAT IS RIDICULOUS! Did you run this through my insurance?

Pharmacist: (*Speaking calmly.*) Yes, ma'am, I did. I understand your frustration, and I am happy to check into this further. It should not take me long but, if you don't mind, please come inside while I resolve this for you. I want to handle this matter promptly as I am sure you are not feeling well and want to get home.

Patient's husband: My wife just got out of the hospital and I just got off work, we are both tired. This is ridiculous how much you are charging us for just two prescriptions.

Pharmacist: I understand your frustration right now, and I want to help you as best as I can. If you can come inside, I will resolve this promptly.

Patient's husband: (*Pauses.*) All right . . . we will drive around and come inside.

(Two minutes later the patient and her husband walk up to the pharmacy counter.)

Patient: Did you figure out the problem? My insurance copay has never been that much. We don't have the money to pay for this right now. I don't get paid until Friday.

Pharmacist: Ms. Brewer, I indeed figured out the issue. Your insurance company has certain medications that they prefer to pay for over others to help reduce their costs. The antibiotic, Levofloxacin, which was prescribed at the hospital, is not on their list of preferred medications, and therefore they are charging you the highest copay, one that you have likely never paid before. Does this make sense?

Patient: So this is not a price that your pharmacy is charging?

Pharmacist: No, we submit the prescription to your insurance company and they provide us with a price. I am happy to call the hospital to suggest a different prescription that your insurance will cover and have them switch to a cheaper alternative.

Patient: That would be great. Thank you.

Pharmacist: Give me a few minutes. I will take care of this promptly.

(The pharmacist leaves the counter to call the insurance company and the hospital while the patient and her husband wait calmly in the waiting room.)

Discussion Questions for the **LEARN** Exercise

1. This chapter suggests that we consider the cognitive, emotional, and behavioral dimensions of conflict. Analyze and discuss the conflict in both patient dialogues by considering these dimensions through the patient's and the pharmacist's perspectives.
2. This text discusses specific strategies to use when trying to resolve conflicts through communication. How did the pharmacist in Dialogue Two use these strategies?
3. As stated in this text, conflicts can quickly become emotionally explosive. The usual advice is to calm the patient in order to make room for a rational conversation. How did the pharmacist respond to the patient's and her husband's emotional state in Dialogue Two?
4. In this case, a misunderstanding on the part of the patient caused the conflict. In a different scenario, if the conflict is caused by more than a simple misunderstanding and you cannot give the patient what he or she wants, what would be your goal in trying to resolve the conflict?

LEARN, PRACTICE, AND ASSESS
CASE STUDY EXERCISES

 PRACTICE: Build Your Own Dialogue

Directions: Now it is time to *practice* what you have learned about the topic of this chapter. Reflecting on concepts from this chapter and the patient dialogues in the LEARN exercise, develop your own pharmacist–patient dialogue using the following patient information and guidance questions.

PATIENT CASE

Gina Green arrives at the pharmacy drive-thru window, driven by her husband, to pick up her prescriptions after leaving the emergency room for the evaluation of injuries suffered during a car accident earlier today. She is groggy and just wants to pick up her prescriptions and go home and go to bed. However, the pharmacy only has one prescription filled, her muscle relaxant Cyclobenzaprine 5 mg BID, instead of both prescriptions called in by the doctor. The nurse did not leave the doctor's Drug Enforcement Administration (DEA) number on the phone message. The doctor cannot be found in the computer system, and although the pharmacist left a message at the hospital, no one has called back with the DEA number. Therefore, the patient's Oxycodone/APAP 5/325 mg is not ready.

As you plan your dialogue, keep in mind what you have learned about communicating with patients about emotionally charged topics. Use the following questions to help plan and assess your dialogue.

1. An important part of planning a dialogue is setting goals for the conversation. Given the patient's situation, what would you like to accomplish in this dialogue? It is good practice to begin with the end in mind. What do you hope the patient will think or feel at the end of your dialogue?

2. How do you plan to accomplish your end goal? Plan your behavioral strategies, both verbal and nonverbal, while considering how the patient and her husband may interpret your behaviors.

3. The patient is groggy and her pain medication is not ready. Consider where a typical patient might place the blame in this situation. How might the patient's misunderstanding about why this happened intensify the conflict? How might you address this misunderstanding?

4. When resolving a conflict, it is important to think about the other party and understand their emotions and their cognitive interpretation of what is happening. What emotions do you think the patient might be

feeling? Cognitively, how might she make sense of what is happening? Plan your dialogue accordingly, given the patient's emotional state and her likely interpretation of the situation.

5. In this chapter, you learned tips on how to manage conflict through communication. Which strategies do you plan to employ during this conversation? Why?

YOUR DIALOGUE HERE

LEARN, PRACTICE, AND ASSESS
CASE STUDY EXERCISES

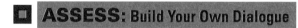
ASSESS: Build Your Own Dialogue

Directions: Now it is time to *assess* what you have learned about the topic of this chapter. In this exercise, no guidance questions are provided. Reflect on what you have learned from the LEARN and PRACTICE exercises, and develop your own pharmacist–patient dialogue using the following patient information.

PATIENT CASE

A 45-year-old female with chronic obstructive pulmonary disease (COPD) and a history of tobacco dependence for 30 years presents to the ambulatory clinic for management of COPD and medication refills. The patient has currently been taking Spiriva 18 mcg daily, Advair 500/50 BID, and Albuterol inhaler prn. The pharmacist consults COPD guidelines for appropriate therapy and discovers that Spiriva and Advair are not recommended to be used in combination to treat COPD. The pharmacist discusses this with the physician, and the physician agrees. The physician discontinues Spiriva, and the patient becomes very upset. The patient states that the pharmacist does not know what he is talking about and she cannot breathe without both inhalers, Spiriva and Advair. The patient uses foul language toward the pharmacist and physician.

YOUR DIALOGUE HERE

DISCUSSION QUESTIONS

1. What school or work-related conflicts have you been involved in recently? Use the concepts in this text to analyze how the parties behaved in the conflicts. What did you learn about communicating in conflict situations from these experiences?
2. Discuss what you think are the most common causes of conflicts between pharmacists and their patients. Which communication strategies do you plan to use when encountering such conflicts?
3. This chapter focuses on conflicts between pharmacists and their patients. Discuss how the principles and strategies presented here may be applied to conflicts between pharmacists and other members of the healthcare team.

REFERENCES

Evans, C. M., Vacca, D., Khanfar, N. M., & Harrington, C. A. (2010). Conflict resolution in a retail community pharmacy: Drugmart Pharmacy case. *Journal of Business Studies Quarterly, 1*(3), 53–67.

Mayer, B. (2012). *The dynamics of conflict: A guide to engagement and intervention* (2nd ed.). San Francisco, CA: Jossey-Bass.

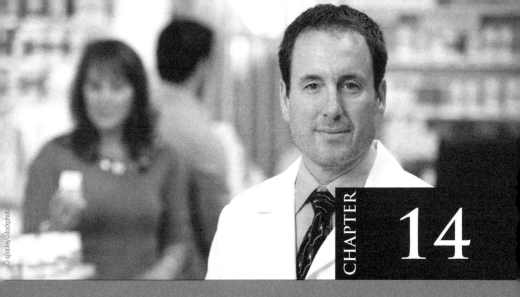

14

PATIENT COMMUNICATION ON SENSITIVE TOPICS

LEARNING OBJECTIVES

At the end of this chapter, students should be able to:

▶ Recognize various types of health issues that may be sensitive topics for patients.

▶ Articulate why certain health issues may be sensitive topics for patients.

▶ Generate communication strategies to provide effective counseling on sensitive health topics.

As healthcare professionals, it is our privilege to serve patients and assist them with their healthcare needs. These needs often manifest as physical or emotional symptoms, and at times patients may find a particular health need or issue difficult to discuss for various reasons. When addressing sensitive issues that patients find difficult to discuss, effective communication skills are essential. Competent patient communication can lead to more patient disclosure of valuable information, better relationships, and improved health outcomes. However, incompetent communication will lead to losing a patient's trust or respect and leave important issues unaddressed. A study by Britto, Tivorsak, and Slap (2010) found that teens of all ages chose not to discuss sensitive topics with providers when they felt the provider would judge them or "jump to conclusions." Some would purposefully avoid a healthcare visit in order to protect their privacy. Handling sensitive topics competently is key to winning the patient's trust.

SENSITIVE HEALTH TOPICS

The online journal *U.S. Pharmacist* published a series of articles concerning communication on such sensitive issues as erectile dysfunction, decreased libido, depression, and menopause (e.g., Berger, 2006). Other sources have identified similar issues that may be sensitive to the patient. Berger (2009) suggests that patients may find it difficult to discuss their concerns about sexual performance, mood disorders, substance abuse, obesity, death and dying, sexual activity and history, domestic violence, psychiatric illness, and alcohol and/or drug abuse.

It is not the purpose of this chapter to generate an exhaustive list of issues toward which pharmacists should display sensitivity. The list is different for each patient and may change over time, even with the same patient. Instead, it is important to understand why such issues are sensitive and difficult for a patient so that you can communicate with the patient in an appropriate manner. Here are some possible explanations:

- *Social stigma associated with health issues.* Given the stigma associated with HIV/AIDS, for instance, HIV patients often prefer to work only with HIV specialty pharmacies because they believe the pharmacists would be more sensitive to their needs (Sherman, 2013).
- *Health conditions that influence the patient's sense of self-worth or identity, including sexual/reproductive health issues.* For instance, some men may find it difficult to discuss erectile dysfunction or male infertility due to such health issues being tied to their sense of masculinity (Berger, 2006).
- *Issues that are considered taboo topics such as death and dying.* With such issues, both the patient and the pharmacist likely have had few opportunities to engage in an open dialogue, which will increase the level of discomfort. The American Society of Health-System Pharmacists (2002) states that the role of the pharmacist in hospice care includes promoting communication, assisting with emotional support, providing education, facilitating access to needed pain medications, and avoiding adverse drug events.

As you consider these possible explanations, think about which topics, if any, tend to make you uncomfortable. If a provider feels discomfort with a certain topic, he or she is less likely to broach the topic or ask the patient questions about it, let alone intentionally engage a patient in what might be a difficult conversation for both parties. For providers, a common reason for not wanting to discuss sensitive topics is the feeling that they are inadequately prepared for the conversation. Planning what you will do, and thinking about specific communication strategies you will use, will help prepare you if and when the conversation arises.

COMMUNICATION STRATEGIES FOR SENSITIVE TOPICS

When communicating with patients on sensitive topics, the pharmacist's ultimate goal is to be caring, supportive, nonjudgmental, and empathic. Here are some specific communication strategies that may be useful:

- Be mindful of subtle *signals* that may indicate patient hesitancy with a topic. Pay attention to any verbal or nonverbal signals that suggest the patient is uncomfortable or anxious.
- Remove *environmental barriers* for communication. If possible, have the conversation in a more private area, and make arrangements so that you have sufficient time and can give the patient your undivided attention.
- Use *verbal and nonverbal tools* to show the patient that you are available and interested in an open conversation. Leaning toward the patient, maintaining good eye contact, asking open-ended questions, and using nonjudgmental language can help the patient feel at ease and make an open conversation more likely.
- Be mindful of one's *own level of comfort* with difficult issues. With topics that make the pharmacist uncomfortable, it is important to remain professional, avoid facial expressions or any other body language that the patient may interpret as judgmental, and focus on understanding the patient's needs. This is important when discussing possible gender-specific issues such as erectile dysfunction or other sexual disorders. If a female pharmacist is discussing erectile dysfunction with a male patient, it is important to remain professional and make the patient feel as comfortable as possible. If you notice that the patient is visibly uncomfortable, offer to have him speak with a male healthcare provider if available.
- *Refrain from giving scripted responses* that may minimize the patient's emotional state. When discussing a sensitive topic, a natural tendency is to resort to scripted responses, such as saying, "I understand your frustration," even when you do not understand. If a patient can see or sense that your response is not genuine, the message will have the opposite effect. Another example is saying, "Don't worry, I am sure you are not alone in having such problems" to a patient sharing her fears over her premenopausal symptoms. Such responses communicate to patients that you are not genuinely interested in understanding their unique emotional state or needs.

Green and Kodish (2009) surveyed more than 400 healthcare providers on communication strategies useful for discussing sensitive topics such as erectile dysfunction with patients. The researchers concluded that there is no one best way to discuss sensitive topics. Instead, the authors argued that it is more important to have critical thinking skills and the ability to comprehend the totality of the situation. Pharmacists must keep in mind the principles of addressing sensitive topics discussed earlier while being cognizant of the uniqueness of each patient and each communication situation.

LEARN, PRACTICE, AND ASSESS
CASE STUDY EXERCISES

● LEARN: Example Patient Dialogues

Directions: Read the following case study. After completing Patient Dialogue One and Patient Dialogue Two, consider the differences between them and answer the questions provided.

PATIENT CASE

John Blankson, a 52-year-old male, has been taking Hydrochlorothiazide 25 mg for high blood pressure for almost 2 months, and he returns to the pharmacy with his prescription bottle for a medication refill. It is around 5:00 p.m. and the retail pharmacy has a line of patients at the prescription intake window. The patient is concerned but also embarrassed about a new problem that has started since he began his high blood pressure medication. The pharmacist is female and is meeting the patient for the first time.

PATIENT DIALOGUE ONE

Pharmacist: Hello, Mr. Blankson. I am Kelly, the pharmacist working today. How are you doing this afternoon?

Patient: Well, I have had better days; thanks for asking.

Pharmacist: (*Taking a look at the prescription bottle and checking patient data in the system.*) I am sorry to hear that. Would you like to get this refilled today?

Patient: Yes. The doctor gave me up to five refills, right?

Pharmacist: Let me see . . . yes, that is correct. You have been taking it for the last month and a half; have you had any problems with the medication? How is your blood pressure?

Patient: Well, I have been taking my blood pressure every day and think the medication is working . . . (*hesitating*) at least in that respect I think it is . . . (*the patient's voice tapers off and he seems concerned*).

Pharmacist: (*The pharmacist fails to notice the patient's uneasiness.*) Well, I am glad that it is! It is important that you continue to take the medication and at the same time monitor your blood pressure every day. We will have your refill ready for you shortly. (*Hands the prescription bottle and the receipt to the patient with a smile.*) Please let us know if you have any questions.

Patient: Well, thanks, I guess. (*The patient walks to the waiting area and contemplates going back to speak with the pharmacist about his concerns but notices she is busy and just waits for his prescription.*)

(Ten minutes later the patient's prescription is ready. He picks it up and leaves with the medication.)

PATIENT DIALOGUE TWO

Pharmacist: Hello, Mr. Blankson. I am Kelly, the pharmacist working today. How are you doing this afternoon?

Patient: Well, I have had better days; thanks for asking.

Pharmacist: (*Stops what she is doing on the computer and looks up at the patient.*) I am sorry to hear that, Mr. Blankson. If there is anything I can do to help, please do not hesitate to let me know.

Patient: (*A few seconds of silence as the patient looks at Kelly and then looks down at his prescription bottle.*) Thank you, I appreciate that. (*He hands the prescription bottle to the pharmacist.*)

Pharmacist: (*The pharmacist takes the prescription bottle from the patient.*) Would you like to get this refilled today?

Patient: Yes. The doctor gave me up to five refills, right?

Pharmacist: Yes, that is correct. I see that you have been taking it for the last month and a half. I'd like to discuss how the medication is working for you. I want to make sure that your blood pressure is under control and that you are not having any problems with the medication.

Patient: Well, I have been taking my blood pressure every day and think the medication is working . . . (*hesitating*) at least in that respect I think it is . . . (*the patient's voice tapers off and he seems concerned*).

Pharmacist: (*The pharmacist notices the patient's uneasiness and leans toward Mr. Blankson.*) I am glad to hear that the medication is working well to keep your blood pressure under control. But I sense that you are not completely satisfied with the medication. Is there anything I can help with?

Patient: (*Hesitating to speak.*) Well, yeah, I guess so. (*An awkward silence; the patient lowers his voice.*) I have been having some issues with my marriage, specifically in the bedroom.

Pharmacist: Mr. Blankson, I want to talk to you about this. Do you mind stepping over here (*pointing to the semi-private patient consultation area*) so that we can discuss this further?

Patient: Sure, no problem. (*He sits down with the pharmacist.*) I see the ads on television and I guess . . . (*struggling to find the right words*) I don't understand why I am having this problem.

Pharmacist: Mr. Blankson, just to make sure I understand, are you experiencing intimacy problems with your spouse?

Patient: (*He nods and seems visibly uncomfortable, hesitating to speak.*) Well . . . yeah. I think I may need Viagra.

Pharmacist: I am glad that you are bringing this to my attention so that we can come to a solution together. There are multiple causes for erectile dysfunction, or ED, and one of them could be the medications you are taking. Patients on this particular blood pressure medication that you are taking have experienced ED, so it is likely that is what is causing the problem.

Patient: (*The patient seems relieved and for the first time looks up at Kelly.*) That's a relief! I wasn't sure if it was my age or something else, and it's never happened to me before. But now that you mention it, the problem started after I began taking this blood pressure pill.

Pharmacist: I would encourage you to discuss this with your doctor. The good news is that your doctor can switch you to a different blood pressure medication.

Patient: Thanks so much! I actually called his office last week but just felt uncomfortable asking about it. I appreciate your talking to me about this.

Pharmacist: You are most welcome. Would you like me to hold off on refilling this prescription until you have a chance to speak with your doctor about your concerns?

Patient: Yes, that'd be great. Thanks so much! (*He seems relieved and satisfied.*)

Pharmacist: My pleasure! Be sure to speak with your doctor as soon as possible so that you don't run out of your medication.

Patient: I will call him as soon as I get in the car. Thanks again.

Discussion Questions for the **LEARN** Exercise

1. As seen in the two patient dialogues, gender can be a factor in a patient's hesitancy to communicate about certain sensitive issues. How did the pharmacist in Dialogue Two, Kelly, help her male patient develop trust in her while discussing a sensitive topic?
2. Pay attention to the verbal and nonverbal strategies Kelly used in Dialogue Two. Did she seem uncomfortable or hesitant at any point in the conversation?
3. The pharmacist in Dialogue One missed the nonverbal cues that the patient was displaying. What do you think are the short- and long-term consequences of this communication fallout?
4. If you were the pharmacist in this case, would you find the topic difficult to discuss with the patient? What additional communication strategies can you think of that might help you communicate with Mr. Blankson?

LEARN, PRACTICE, AND ASSESS
CASE STUDY EXERCISES

 PRACTICE: Build Your Own Dialogue

Directions: Now it is time to *practice* what you have learned about the topic of this chapter. Reflecting on concepts from this chapter and the patient dialogues in the LEARN exercise, develop your own pharmacist–patient dialogue using the following patient information and guidance questions.

PATIENT CASE

James Richards is a 64-year-old man with stage IV colon cancer (the last stage that continues to spread to multiple organs and areas of the body) who was admitted to the hospital with severe abdominal pain and distention and nausea with vomiting. In the emergency room he was immediately given medications to help his symptoms and diagnostic tests were performed. Imaging scans showed widespread tumors throughout the liver and new tumors in his lungs. The patient has received multiple prior chemotherapy regimens. The oncologist informed the patient that he has a very poor prognosis, recommended no further chemotherapy be given, and suggested the patient consider hospice care. The pharmacist is asked to discuss medications that the patient can still take while receiving hospice care that will make him comfortable, including morphine for pain, Lorazepam for anxiety, and Compazine for nausea. The patient and family are nervous about discontinuing chemotherapy, and the patient is scared of dying.

As you plan your dialogue, keep in mind what you have learned about discussing sensitive topics with patients. Use the following questions to help plan and assess your dialogue.

1. An important part of planning a dialogue is setting goals for the conversation. Given the patient's and the family's situation, what would you like to accomplish in this dialogue? Be sure to think about both short- and long-term goals. For instance, you may want to comfort the patient and his fears of dying by offering to call a chaplain to the room, discuss any concerns that the patient and the family may have, and help them understand how palliative care works. However, a more important goal may be to communicate to the patient and family that you want to answer any questions they have, help the patient feel as comfortable as possible, and listen to what they have to say.

2. It is good practice to begin with the end in mind. What do you hope the patient will think or feel at the end of your dialogue? How do you plan to accomplish this?

3. A general rule is that if you have never personally gone through this situation, it is better to avoid giving scripted responses such as "I understand." What other responses do you want to avoid during this dialogue?
4. This may be the first time the pharmacist is speaking with the patient. If so, a level of discomfort exists, and the patient and family are in need of emotional support. This is an important time to display empathy and interest. How will you verbally and nonverbally display empathy and interest?

YOUR DIALOGUE HERE

LEARN, PRACTICE, AND ASSESS
CASE STUDY EXERCISES

 ASSESS: Build Your Own Dialogue

Directions: Now it is time to *assess* what you have learned about the topic of this chapter. In this exercise, no guidance questions are provided. Reflect on what you have learned from the LEARN and PRACTICE exercises, and develop your own pharmacist–patient dialogue using the following patient information.

PATIENT CASE

Tracy Jones is a 22-year-old female who was recently diagnosed with HIV. She had been in a heterosexual relationship for the past 2 years when she found out that her boyfriend was cheating on her. She is distraught and very embarrassed to pick up her new prescription. She has questions about the medication COMPLERA (emtricitabine/rilpivirine/tenofovir disoproxil fumarate), but she wants privacy and wants to speak only with the pharmacist.

YOUR DIALOGUE HERE

DISCUSSION QUESTIONS

1. Ask someone who knows you well to find out which verbal and non-verbal cues you tend to display when discussing a topic that makes you uncomfortable. How might those cues affect your communication with a patient about a sensitive health topic?
2. This text discusses a range of topics that can be sensitive to patients. Consider which topics tend to make you uncomfortable. Discuss specific strategies you plan to use if these topics need to be discussed with a patient.
3. Depending on your age, gender, ethnicity, and other characteristics, some patients may find it more or less difficult to discuss their sensitive health needs with you. An older male patient may be uncomfortable discussing his bladder issues with a young female pharmacist, compared to someone who is older and of the same sex. How might you help make the patient in this or a similar situation more comfortable?
4. Consider the physical environment at your pharmacy or organization. What changes can be made to make patients more comfortable when discussing sensitive health topics?

REFERENCES

American Society of Health-System Pharmacists. (2002). ASHP statement on the pharmacist's role in hospice and palliative care. *American Journal of Health-Systems Pharmacists, 59,* 1770–1773.

Berger, B. A. (2006). Communication concerning sensitive issues: Counseling on erectile dysfunction. *U.S. Pharmacist, 8,* 96–102.

Berger, B. A. (2009). *Communication skills for pharmacists: Building relationships, improving patient care* (3rd ed.). Washington, DC: American Pharmacists Association.

Britto, M. T., Tivorsak, T. L., & Slap, G. B. (2010). Adolescents' needs for health care privacy. *Pediatrics, 126*(6), e1469–e1476. doi:10.1542/peds.2010-0389

Green, R., & Kodish, S. (2009). Discussing a sensitive topic: Nurse practitioners' and physician assistants' communication strategies in managing patients with erectile dysfunction. *Journal of the American Academy of Nurse Practitioners, 21*(12), 698–705.

Sherman, M. J. (2013, February 13). Know your pharmacist, know your pharmacy. *Thebody.com.* Retrieved from http://www.thebody.com/content/70261/know-your-pharmacist-know-your-pharmacy.html

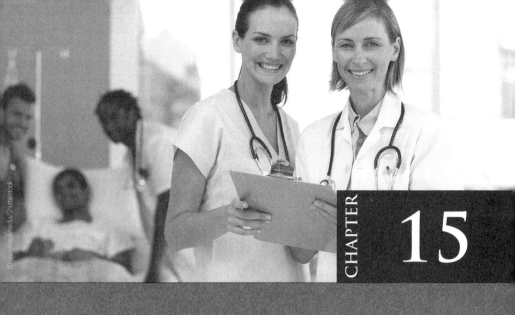

15

INTERPROFESSIONAL COMMUNICATION

LEARNING OBJECTIVES

At the end of this chapter, students should be able to:

▸ Recognize the importance of interprofessional collaboration.
▸ Define interprofessional communication and recognize its importance in interprofessional collaboration.
▸ Identify common barriers to interprofessonal communication.
▸ Identify communication strategies, including various sources of power, to achieve effective interprofessional communication.

KEY TERMS

Coercive power

Expertise power

Information power

Interprofessional collaboration

Interprofessional communication

Legitimate power

Reward power

Consider the number of times you have collaborated with others to complete a team project during your professional education. Chances are that in your educational experience you have had to work with others as a team. During your professional program, have you had an opportunity to work in teams with those learning to be a physician, nurse, dentist, or other healthcare providers? If your answer is no, you are not alone. A 2011 report by the Robert Wood Johnson Foundation notes that most U.S. healthcare providers have not been trained to work as part of integrated teams. Lack of training in this area explains why many healthcare providers do not have the skills to collaborate with others regarding patient care. **Interprofessional collaboration**, which is collaboration among members from different professions, can be particularly challenging in healthcare settings.

Research has long suggested that interprofessional collaboration improves coordination, communication, and, ultimately, the quality and safety of patient care. Pharmacists as well as other professionals, such as physicians and nurses, all recognize, at least in principle, the importance of working as a team for delivering optimum patient care. The World Health Organization (2010) also calls for a more collaborative approach to promoting individual and public health. Collaborative practice happens when multiple health professionals from different professional backgrounds work together with patients, families, and communities to deliver the highest quality of care.

The Center for the Advancement of Pharmacy Education's 2013 educational outcomes clearly identify interprofessional collaboration as a core competency for pharmacy students (Medina et al., 2013). Students should be able to actively participate in interprofessional collaboration and engage other healthcare team members by demonstrating mutual respect, understanding, and values to meet patient care needs. The outcomes also identified specific learning objectives that pharmacy students should meet in regard to interprofessional collaboration:

- Establish a climate of shared values and mutual respect necessary to meet patient care needs.
- Define clear roles and responsibilities for team members to optimize outcomes for specific patient care encounters.
- Communicate in a manner that values team-based decision making and shows respect for contributions from other areas of expertise.
- Foster accountability and leverage expertise to form a highly functioning team (one that includes the patient, family, and community) and promote shared patient-centered problem solving.

DEFINING INTERPROFESSIONAL COMMUNICATION

Competent communication with all members of the healthcare team while caring for patients is key to the success of interprofessional collaboration. **Interprofessional communication** occurs when members of the healthcare team communicate in a collaborative manner for information exchange, collaborative decision making, and ultimately for attaining optimum patient outcomes.

Interprofessional communication may differ in meaning, depending on where the pharmacist practices. In hospital and ambulatory care settings, this may entail participating in patient rounds, providing medication reconciliation and therapeutic monitoring, and being a part of the patient education and discharge process. In the community pharmacy setting, more of the interprofessional communication will take place on the phone or via electronic methods of communication.

IMPORTANCE OF INTERPROFESSIONAL COMMUNICATION

The benefits of interprofessional collaborations to patient care are well established. Patients report higher levels of satisfaction, better adherence, and improved health outcomes following treatment delivered with a collaborative team approach (O'Daniel & Rosenstein, 2008). Researchers have also shown that competent interprofessional communication among healthcare teams can lead to a decrease in patient complications, shorter and fewer hospital stays, and a reduction in conflict among caregivers and in staff turnover. On the other hand, poor interprofessional communication and lack of team collaboration can be very costly. A 2011 report by the Robert Wood Johnson Foundation argues that the lack of quality collaboration among different healthcare providers is partly to blame for why the U.S. healthcare system is so costly and fraught with errors.

BARRIERS TO INTERPROFESSIONAL COMMUNICATION

Barriers that make everyday teamwork difficult also apply to interprofessional patient care teams. *Individual-level barriers* include different personal values and expectations, lack of experience working in teams, and personality clashes. More barriers function at the *institutional* and *professional levels* as well.

Healthcare professionals can display territorial actions when working with other healthcare providers. A nurse may feel that pharmacists should stick to dispensing medications and not provide immunizations, even if allowed by the state law. Pharmacists may feel that they can obtain vitals and disregard the use of a nurse. Among the different healthcare professions, there are variations in professional standards and protocols, language and jargon, and educational experience and background, all of which make collaboration more challenging. However, these differences among professions can also make interprofessional communication even more important and rewarding.

The potential influence of historical interprofessional rivalries on interprofessional communication and collaboration is worth considering. Throughout your experience as a pharmacy student, you may have been exposed to discussions that emphasize how different professions, such as medicine, nursing, and pharmacy, have varying levels of preparation, which gives the professionals different levels of expertise and status. Rivalry also exists beyond the interpersonal level. A recent example occurred in 2013 when the American Medical Association House of Delegates adopted a resolution calling inquiries from pharmacies about the rationale behind prescriptions, diagnoses, and treatment plans to be an "interference with the practice of medicine and unwarranted" (National Association of Boards of Pharmacy, 2013). Pharmacy professionals' reactions to this varied, but most would agree that such a resolution would affect physician–pharmacist interactions and collaborations. As you find yourself communicating with others as part of a healthcare team, consider debates or rivalries such as these in the context of your communication with those from other professions and keep in mind how it may affect one's preconceived view of the pharmacy profession.

PHARMACIST COMMUNICATION GOALS IN INTERPROFESSIONAL TEAMS

As discussed in the chapter on Pharmacy Patient Communication, daily communication may serve *functional goals,* such as providing information or persuading someone, and *relational goals,* such as relieving tension or establishing trust (McCornack, 2009). Similarly, while working in interprofessional teams, a pharmacist's communication goals may include informing, persuading, building relationships, or establishing expertise and trust. In most cases, you will find yourself working on multiple goals simultaneously. As you read the following communication scenarios, consider the pharmacist's specific *communication goals* and identify any *barriers* that may be encountered:

- After graduation, you start working at a hospital and become a part of the inpatient internal medicine team. You notice that the attending physicians never ask for your input on medications. They are older and may not be used to having pharmacists on the medical team.

Overhearing their conversations, you realize that they seem unaware of how much training is required for pharmacists and the breadth of knowledge and drug expertise that a pharmacist can contribute.

- When a patient comes in with a prescription for a statin medication, you ask if she is experiencing any side effects. The patient mentions some recent memory loss. You know that memory loss is a side effect of the particular statin drug the patient is taking. You would like to recommend another statin drug to her doctor but realize that the physician seems to have always prescribed that particular statin drug.

- Working as a community pharmacist, your job routinely involves medication reconciliation. You become concerned with possible drug interactions regarding a new medication prescribed by a physician to your patient. You want to ask the doctor to reconsider, but you also know that this doctor is busy and does not always have the patience for this kind of consultation.

HOW TO HAVE A VOICE ON INTERPROFESSIONAL TEAMS

While communicating with other healthcare professionals, your success depends on your ability to negotiate and exert confidence and influence through your knowledge and expertise for the overall goal of improving patient outcomes. Scholars such as French and Raven (1959) have identified different sources of power that are relevant to pharmacists working in interprofessional settings. **Expertise power** refers to one's ability to influence others based on specific skills or knowledge. This is slightly different from **legitimate power**, which refers to authority associated with a position or one's title. **Information power** is the possession of or access to information that others perceive as valuable. There is also **reward power**, which comes with one's ability to give positive benefits, and **coercive power**, which comes with the power to punish or control.

As you engage in interprofessional communication, consider the type of power or influence that each party brings to the conversation and how you can utilize different sources of power to advocate for your position. Consider the three different scenarios presented earlier. How might you use different sources of power to accomplish your communication goals in each case?

It is also important to remember that individuals' perception of power and influence may differ, which will also shape the conversation. Given physicians' legal authority to prescribe medications, they are typically perceived as possessing more power, specifically *legitimate power*. As a pharmacist, you may rely on your training and try to exert your *expertise power* when interacting with a physician. However, your ability to accomplish that goal may ultimately depend on your ability to persuade the physician to recognize and trust your expertise. In order to accomplish this, communication is key. Developing collaborative working relationships with physicians is in the best interest of patients; however, there is no guarantee that the pharmacist's effort will be reciprocated, and in some cases, the process could be a difficult one (McDonough & Doucette, 2001).

Ultimately, a pharmacist's goal is to be an advocate for the patient's health, a goal with which all healthcare professionals identify. This common ground of shared interest and goals can be used to address any barriers or challenges in interprofessional communication.

LEARN, PRACTICE, AND ASSESS
CASE STUDY EXERCISES

LEARN: Example Patient Dialogues

Directions: Read the following case study. After completing Patient Dialogue One and Patient Dialogue Two, consider the differences between them and answer the questions provided.

PATIENT CASE

Margaret Green, a 45-year-old woman, presents to a primary care clinic consisting of physicians, nurse practitioners, nurses, counselors, and a clinical pharmacist. Each healthcare professional sees patients individually. The clinical pharmacist is new to the clinic and has recently started providing medication management services. The addition of this new pharmacy service has caused tension in the clinic due to territorial feelings by most healthcare providers. The pharmacist is seeing this patient for the first time for medication management services. Her current medications include:

* Benicar 20 mg 1 tablet by mouth daily
* OTC women's multivitamin 1 tablet by mouth daily

PATIENT DIALOGUE ONE

Pharmacist: Hello, Ms. Green. I am Gina, the pharmacist, and I will be going over your medications with you today.

Patient: Okay. Am I not seeing my doctor today?

Pharmacist: Not today. I am going to check your vitals and make sure you are on the best medications and that there are no interactions or problems with your medications.

(The patient apprehensively walks back to the office with the pharmacist.)

Pharmacist: Please have a seat and I will check your blood pressure.

(The pharmacist checks the patient's blood pressure, which is 188/98, and obtains a medication list and history from the patient.)

Pharmacist: Wow, I can't believe your doctor only has you on Benicar 20 mg daily for your blood pressure. I will make a recommendation for your doctor to increase your dose and add on a water pill.

(The pharmacist inputs the recommendations in the electronic medical record for the patient's physician. The patient's physician sees the recommendations and ignores them. Instead of increasing the Benicar to 40 mg, he adds on HCTZ 12.5 mg to Benicar 20 mg. The pharmacist gets upset and approaches the physician.)

Pharmacist: (*Talking to the physician.*) Did you see my recommendations for Ms. Green?

Physician: Yes, I did, but I chose to add on a diuretic instead of increasing the Benicar.

Pharmacist: Okay. (*Walks away upset.*)

PATIENT DIALOGUE TWO

Pharmacist: Hello, Ms. Green. I am Gina, the pharmacist, and I will be going over your medications with you today.

Patient: Okay. Am I not seeing my doctor today?

Pharmacist: Not today. I am going to check your vitals and make sure you are on the best medications and that there are no interactions or problems with your medications.

(The patient apprehensively walks back to the office with the pharmacist.)

Pharmacist: Please have a seat and I will check your blood pressure.

(The pharmacist checks the patient's blood pressure, which is 188/98, and obtains a medication list and history from the patient.)

Pharmacist: Ms. Green, your blood pressure is high today. When was the last time you took your medication?

Patient: I took my medication with my vitamin this morning like I do every morning.

Pharmacist: Okay, great. Well, your blood pressure is high today, but we can lower it by increasing your blood pressure pill. I will discuss this with your doctor and follow up with you by phone.

(The pharmacist inputs a medication increase recommendation in the electronic medical record for the patient's physician. She includes a justification of optimizing one medication before adding another medication. The physician sees the recommendation and ignores it. Instead of increasing the Benicar, the doctor adds on HCTZ 12.5 mg daily. The pharmacist chooses to discuss the recommendation with the physician in person.)

Pharmacist: Hello, Dr. Lamb. Do you have a few minutes to discuss the recommendations I provided for Ms. Margaret Green's blood pressure?

Physician: Um, if you can make it quick. I have another patient to see.

Pharmacist: (*Smiling with a pleasant demeanor.*) Sure, I will make it quick. Ms. Green's blood pressure was high today at 188/98, which is well above her goal of 140/90, according to the JNC 8 guidelines. It is recommended to optimize one medication before adding another medication. The Benicar can be increased to 40 mg daily. Adding HCTZ will result in her having to take two pills instead of one for her blood pressure. If her blood pressure is still not controlled on the Benicar 40 mg, it would be ideal to then add on HCTZ and a combination Benicar HCT is available.

Physician: Okay (*pauses*) . . . that makes sense. I will make the change and have the clerk contact her about the medication change.

Pharmacist: Okay, great. I would be glad to call her to discuss this change.

Physician: Okay, thanks.

Discussion Questions for the **LEARN** Exercise

1. The patient's well-being should always be the priority when providing care. Consider Dialogue One; in what ways might patient-centered care be compromised in that case?
2. How did the pharmacist exert her expertise power in Dialogue Two during the interaction with the physician? Which other sources of power could the pharmacist use while communicating with other members of the healthcare team?
3. What if, at the end of Dialogue Two, the physician still seems unwilling to follow your recommendation? Discuss additional communication skills or strategies that pharmacists in similar situations can utilize to help persuade the physician while also gaining his or her respect.

LEARN, PRACTICE, AND ASSESS ● ▲ ▢
CASE STUDY EXERCISES

 PRACTICE: Build Your Own Dialogue

Directions: Now it is time to *practice* what you have learned about the topic of this chapter. Reflecting on concepts from this chapter and the patient dialogues in the LEARN exercise, develop your own pharmacist–patient dialogue using the following patient information and guidance questions.

PATIENT CASE

Justin Bedell, a 57-year-old male, has newly diagnosed hypertension in addition to type 2 diabetes, for which he takes Metformin 1000 mg BID and Glimeperide 4 mg daily. He was started on Metoprolol Succinate 100 mg daily for hypertension with no compelling indication for a beta blocker. Mr. Bedell comes to the clinic to see the pharmacist for the first time and his vitals are as follows:

* Blood pressure = 150/88
* Pulse = 60

The pharmacist will provide appropriate recommendations to the patient's physician to optimize medication therapy and improve patient outcomes.

As you plan your dialogue, keep in mind what you have learned about interprofessional communication. Use the following questions to help plan and assess your dialogue.

1. To promote interprofessional collaboration, it is important to communicate in a manner that values team-based decision making and shows respect for other healthcare professionals. How can you do this when discussing the drug-related problem (DRP)—drug with no indication—with the patient's physician?
2. What potential communication problems or conflicts may arise during communication with the physician? Consider verbal and nonverbal communication that could create communication barriers.
3. What could be prevented if the DRP is addressed and corrected? How can you communicate the importance of this DRP in a nonthreatening manner?
4. There are five types of power relevant to pharmacists working in interprofessional settings: expertise power, legitimate power, information power, reward power, and coercive power. Which type(s) of power do you plan to utilize in your dialogue with the patient's physician? Why?

YOUR DIALOGUE HERE

LEARN, PRACTICE, AND ASSESS
CASE STUDY EXERCISES

ASSESS: Build Your Own Dialogue

Directions: Now it is time to *assess* what you have learned about the topic of this chapter. In this exercise, no guidance questions are provided. Reflect on what you have learned from the LEARN and PRACTICE exercises, and develop your own pharmacist–patient dialogue using the following patient information.

PATIENT CASE

James Foster is a 39-year-old male with a history of type 2 diabetes, hypertension, asthma, and obesity. He smokes one pack of cigarettes per day. His calculated ASCVD risk is 18%. The patient's lipid panel is as follows: TC 242; LDL 113; TG 348; HDL 32. According to the new lipid guidelines, the patient is indicated for a high-intensity statin. The patient presents to the clinic for follow up with the clinical pharmacist and endocrinologist. The pharmacist recommends starting Crestor 20 mg daily. The endocrinologist does not fully accept the new lipid guidelines and feels that the patient does not need to be on such a high-dose statin, especially with his LDL "being so low." The pharmacist and the endocrinologist have a face-to-face meeting to discuss the recommendation further.

YOUR DIALOGUE HERE

DISCUSSION QUESTIONS

1. As discussed in this text and illustrated in the patient cases, physicians may display territorial actions by consciously choosing to ignore the pharmacist's recommendations. Discuss specific services or scenarios where healthcare providers may display territorial actions.
2. What are the possible implications of territorial thinking in an interprofessional practice environment?
3. What opportunities have you had to interact and collaborate with health professionals of different professions? What has your experience been like?
4. This text discusses barriers that might make collaborative teamwork difficult in patient care. Which barriers have you observed or noticed? What do you think is a pharmacist's role in promoting interprofessional collaboration while caring for patients?

REFERENCES

French, J. R. P., & Raven, B. (1959). The bases of social power. In D. Cartwright (Ed.), *Studies in social power* (pp. 150–167). Ann Arbor, MI: Institute for Social Research, University of Michigan.

McCornack, S. (2009). *Reflect and relate: An introduction to interpersonal communication* (2nd ed.). Boston, MA: Bedford/St. Martin's.

McDonough, R. P., & Doucette, W. R. (2001). Dynamics of pharmaceutical care: Developing collaborative working relationships between pharmacists and physicians. *Journal of the American Pharmacists Association, 41*(5), 682–692.

Medina, M. S., Plaza, C. M., Stowe, C. D., Robinson, E. T., DeLander, G., Beck, D. E., … Johnston, P. (2013). Center for the Advancement of Pharmacy Education 2013 educational outcomes. *American Journal of Pharmaceutical Education, 77*(8), 162. doi:10.5688/ajpe778162

National Association of Boards of Pharmacy. (2013, July 3). *AMA policy deems "inappropriate queries" from pharmacists an interference with practice of medicine* [News release]. Retrieved from http://www.nabp.net/news/ama-policy-deems-inappropriate-queries-from-pharmacies-an-interference-with-practice-of-medicine

O'Daniel, M., & Rosenstein, A. H. (2008). Chapter 33: Professional communication and team collaboration. In R. G. Hughes (Ed.), *Patient safety and quality: An evidence-based handbook for nurses*. Rockville, MD: Agency for Healthcare Research and Quality. Retrieved from http://www.ncbi.nlm.nih.gov/books/NBK2637/

Robert Wood Johnson Foundation. (2011, September). What can be done to encourage more interprofessional collaboration in health care? *Health Policy Snapshot*. Retrieved from http://www.rwjf.org/content/dam/farm/reports/issue_briefs/2011/rwjf72058

World Health Organization. (2010). *Framework for action on interprofessional education and collaborative practice*. Geneva, Switzerland: Author.

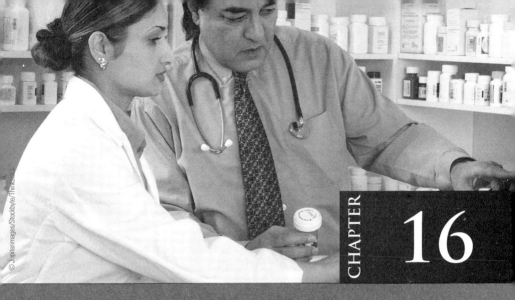

CHAPTER

16

PHARMACY COMMUNICATION IN DIVERSE SETTINGS

LEARNING OBJECTIVES

At the end of this chapter, students should be able to:

▸ Identify the diverse professional settings in which pharmacists practice.

▸ Explain how the professional setting may define what competent pharmacy communication entails.

▸ Articulate ways in which communication technologies shape patient communication.

In 2012, more than 12,000 students graduated with a PharmD degree and entered the profession of pharmacy, a number that is estimated to exceed 14,000 by 2016 (American Association of Colleges of Pharmacy, 2013). According to statistics from 2006, about 62% of those graduates will be working in community pharmacies, approximately 23% in hospitals, and the remainder in nontraditional settings (Council on Credentialing in Pharmacy, 2009). No matter which setting one works in, a pharmacist's daily practice will require communication skills. These include patient education, motivational interviewing, and information exchange with patients, caregivers, insurers and other payers, and other healthcare professionals. However, diverse practice settings may also present unique challenges for communication.

As discussed in the chapter on Pharmacy Patient Communication, competent communication requires one to be *effective* in achieving communication goals and to be *appropriate* and *ethical* while achieving those goals (McCornack, 2009). Consider the communication goal of convincing a patient that she needs to make certain lifestyle changes in addition to taking certain medications. What it takes to effectively achieve this goal depends greatly on such patient characteristics as their health needs. It also depends on the location of the conversation—whether it is in a hospital setting when the medication is prescribed or at a community setting where filling of the prescription is taking place. In other words, to achieve effective, appropriate, and ethical communication, pharmacy professionals must be cognizant of the setting in which they are practicing and any unique situational demands present in the setting.

DOMAINS OF PHARMACY PRACTICE

Consider the different professional practice settings in which a pharmacist may work. The Council on Credentialing in Pharmacy (2009) proposed a three-dimensional model that encompasses the three major domains of pharmacy practice: *patient care, systems management,* and *public health.* In the patient care domain of pharmacy practice, pharmacists are involved in direct patient care in various settings ranging from community pharmacy to hospital settings. In this domain are hospital pharmacists, clinical pharmacists, advanced generalist practitioners, or advanced focused practitioners. Generalist practitioners work in community pharmacies, hospitals, and ambulatory care clinics, and they serve the bulk of pharmacy patient needs in their settings. Focused practitioners serve a specific patient population and often work in specialized settings, such as pediatrics or geriatrics. Advanced generalist practitioners provide services to a wide variety of patients with complex healthcare issues covering a broad range of diseases and could include pharmacists who are board certified in a broader specialty such as pharmacotherapy. Advanced focused practitioners specialize in narrow, focused patient populations with complicated healthcare needs, such as HIV/AIDS patients, oncology patients, and psychiatric patients. These examples of generalist practitioners show a broader patient and practice focus compared to the more specific areas of focused practitioners. Advanced-level practitioners require more advanced levels of knowledge, skills, and experiences compared to generalists.

COMMUNITY PHARMACY
VERSUS HOSPITAL PHARMACY

The majority of patient needs for pharmacy services are met by generalist practitioners, so let us focus on this specific group of professionals. Within this category exists much diversity regarding the specific patient care setting.

Someone working in a community pharmacy setting will face different communication challenges compared to someone working in a hospital. One concern for pharmacy communication in hospital settings is, for instance, reducing medication errors, specifically dispensing errors (Cheung, Bouvy, & De Smet, 2009), which refer to discrepancies between a prescription and the medicine that the pharmacy delivers to the patient or the ward. Hospital pharmacies typically serve patients with more acute health needs and for each patient may collaborate with a different set of healthcare professionals. This creates more challenges for communication. The Agency for Healthcare Research and Quality (2003) identified communication problems as a leading cause of medication errors, which further emphasizes the importance of effective communication for hospital pharmacists to achieve safe and effective patient care.

In the hospital setting, a pharmacist has access to a variety of tools and resources that facilitate communication and collaboration, including communication technologies (such as pagers, portable phones, and tablet computers), patient data management systems (such as electronic medical records), and routine patient rounds. There are also checkpoint systems put in place to reduce communication breakdown and ensure accurate flow of information. In a community setting, pharmacists most likely do not have access to these tools or resources to facilitate the continuity of care for each patient. Hence, they may find themselves struggling more with care fragmentation, incomplete medical records, nonadherence, and other preventable patient care errors. These issues can be seen as communication problems or challenges, and to address them, innovative approaches are needed to improve communication. In one study, discharged patients with an average of five prescriptions were given a one-page pharmacy-to-pharmacy referral form detailing diagnosis, medication regimen, medication history, drug allergies, and other relevant information; the patient's pharmacy received a copy also (Wick, 2006). The majority of the pharmacist participants reported that this simple summary allowed them to focus on counseling and to maintain an updated record for their patients.

COMMUNICATION AND INFORMATION TECHNOLOGIES

Technological advances have created tools that can make communication more convenient, efficient, and timely. Community pharmacy chains such as CVS and Walgreens have invested for years in mobile communication tools such as apps for managing multiple prescriptions and in having customizable health and medication news feeds delivered to the patient's smartphone (Johnson, 2013). Electronic prescribing allows a prescriber to "electronically send an accurate, error-free and understandable prescription directly to a pharmacy" (Nosta, 2013), an important tool for reducing dispensing errors and improving patient safety. Another ongoing national movement toward e-health is the use of electronic health records (EHR), a movement in which pharmacists are expected to play a significant role, particularly in using EHRs in transitions of care and medication reconciliation (Pharmacy e-Health Information Technology Collaborative, 2011).

As different professions continue to invest in the next newest communication technology, it is important to keep in mind that the fundamental goals and principles of pharmacist–patient communication still apply, no matter how technologically advanced our communication becomes. Whether we are sending reminders to patients via postal mail, text message, or email, the goal remains the same: to increase patient outcomes by improving adherence to medication therapy. In communicating with patients face-to-face, on the phone, using social networking sites, or via email, our focus will always be on building relationships, maintaining open communication, and increasing understanding. It is also important to remain professional no matter which form of communication is being used. The use of technology for communication can easily lead to miscommunication due to the lack of nonverbal cues such as facial expressions. Therefore, extra effort, such as choosing your words appropriately and avoiding spelling errors, must be made when communicating via text message, Facebook, or Twitter.

The founder of a health information technology company specializing in digitally connecting patients to pharmacists stated, "our goal is to empower them [pharmacists] with the tools to extend their real-world patient relationships into the digital landscape" (Nosta, 2013). As patients become more consumed by the digital world and spend more time with online communication media and social networking sites, healthcare professionals—including pharmacists—must continuously assess their patients' communication needs and reinvent their communication strategies.

REFERENCES

Agency for Healthcare Research and Quality. (2003). *ARHQ's patient safety initiative: Building foundations, reducing risk.* Retrieved from http://www.ahrq.gov/research/findings/final-reports/pscongrpt/psini2.html

American Association of Colleges of Pharmacy. (2013). *Profile of pharmacy students: Fall 2012.* Alexandria, VA: Author.

Cheung, K. C., Bouvy, M. L., & De Smet, P. A. (2009). Medication errors: The importance of safe dispensing. *British Journal of Clinical Pharmacology, 67*(6), 676–680.

Council on Credentialing in Pharmacy. (2009). *Scope of contemporary pharmacy practice: Roles, responsibilities, and functions of pharmacists and pharmacy technicians.* Washington, DC: Author.

Johnson, L. (2013, July 2). CVS/pharmacy aims for more comprehensive mobile tool via app update. *Mobile Commerce Daily*. Retrieved from http://www.mobilecommercedaily.com/cvspharmacy-aims-for-more-comprehensive-mobile-tool-via-app-update

McCornack, S. (2009). *Reflect and relate: An introduction to interpersonal communication* (2nd ed.). Boston, MA: Bedford/St. Martin's.

Nosta, J. (2013, August 20). Digital health and the pharmacy: A prescription for success. *Forbes*. Retrieved from http://www.forbes.com/sites/johnnosta/2013/08/20/digital-health-and-the-pharmacy-a-prescription-for-success/

Pharmacy e-Health Information Technology Collaborative. (2011). *The roadmap for pharmacy health information technology integration in U.S. health care*. Retrieved from https://www.accp.com/docs/positions/misc/HITRoadMap2011.pdf

Wick, J. Y. (2006, May 1). Broadening pharmacy's role: Continuity of care. *Pharmacy Times*. Retrieved from http://www.pharmacytimes.com/publications/issue/2006/2006-05/2006-05-5537

EPILOGUE

Congratulations! You have made it to the end of this text! For pharmacists, the skill of communication is an essential tool for understanding and serving patient needs, collaborating effectively with colleagues, achieving optimum patient care outcomes, and establishing and maintaining meaningful relationships, personal or professional.

A JOURNEY TOWARD COMMUNICATION COMPETENCY

Even though you have reached the end of this text on pharmacy communication, your journey to becoming a competent communicator has just begun. When it comes to building communication competence, all of us should take a *lifelong learning* approach. Communication is always evolving. You have likely heard the saying that one can never step into the same river twice. Following the same logic, you can never have the same communication encounter twice. This ever-changing nature of communication is what makes it exciting, but it also means that every day you will find yourself facing new challenges and learning new skills as a communicator. Instead of thinking of communication competency as a destination that you can finally "arrive at" one day, we encourage you to focus on constantly refining your communication skills and mindfully applying those skills to different communication situations in the most competent way.

A MODEL OF COMMUNICATION COMPETENCE

In his book *Empathic Communication* (1986), William Howell presented a model of communication competence that included four levels: unconscious incompetence, conscious incompetence, conscious competence, and unconscious competence. This model (see **Figure 1**) is a useful tool when reflecting on how to best build skills such as communication.

You may know someone who is rude or offensive while communicating with others and have wondered whether the individual knows he or she is being rude and offensive. When someone is being incompetent as a communicator and is unaware of it, they are at *Level One*. Change or learning is unlikely to happen until one moves to *Level Two*. Think back to the time when you were learning to drive a car or speak a foreign language. Whomever was teaching you likely kept reminding you of the right way to drive or to speak, while you continued to make mistakes. When we make mistakes but are aware of our incompetence, we are at Level Two. As you can see, moving from Level One to Level Two is a key step toward building your competency as a communicator. A key difference between the two steps is that, at Level Two, one is being conscious and mindful of what is appropriate and effective. As you contemplate the first two levels of communication competence, consider the following questions:

- Individuals at Level One are unaware that they are at that level. Think about your own communication. Could you be unconsciously incompetent with communication? If so, would you want someone to tell you? Would you tell a friend who is at that level?

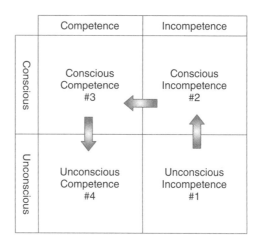

	Competence	Incompetence
Conscious	Conscious Competence #3	Conscious Incompetence #2
Unconscious	Unconscious Competence #4	Unconscious Incompetence #1

Figure 1   Four levels of communication competence.

- What are some areas in which you are currently consciously incompetent? What are you doing to improve and move to the next level?

At *Level Three*, we have communicators who are consciously competent. They are being appropriate, effective, and ethical in their communication with others, make a conscious effort at being competent, and are mindful of their actions and the communication process. Think back to the last time you had a big interview, such as an interview for a job or even an interview for admission into pharmacy school, or needed to have an important talk with a relational partner. You likely strategically planned for the encounter and thought about how you would present yourself and your ideas in the most effective way. As a result of this effort, you hoped to achieve communication that was appropriate, effective, and ethical. By being mindful and making a conscious effort, we become more competent with our communication.

Chances are that many of our daily communication will not require the same kind of strategic planning or conscious effort as does an interview. When you greet a patient with a smile, look him or her in the eye, and nod and listen with empathy as an emotional patient talks, you likely do this without giving much thought to why or how you are doing it. This is an example of *Level Four*, where we are unconsciously competent in our communication. Sometimes it is referred to as being on *autopilot*. With low-demand, routine communication, one can be in an autopilot mode, which requires less mental effort and allows us to be effective and efficient. However, when in high-demand communication situations, such as serving a limited English proficiency patient or communicating about a sensitive topic, we should switch to Level Three and make a conscious effort to choose the most appropriate communication strategies for the patient and the situation. Reflect on the following questions regarding Level Three and Level Four:

- Some argue that when we believe ourselves to be unconsciously competent at something, we risk being complacent and could slip back to Level One, unconscious incompetence, without our knowledge. What do you think?
- Many of the chapters focused on communication situations considered to be high demand, such as emotionally charged communication. What other communication situations do you personally consider to be high demand, requiring you to be in Level Three?

When encountering a new and unfamiliar communication task, you will probably start in Level One or Level Two. The goal is to build competence and reach Level Three or Level Four through reflection, practice, and repetition, as we have encouraged you to do throughout this text.

CONCLUDING THOUGHTS

Communication is a learnable skill and one that we can acquire only through a repetition of practice and reflection. As you embark on this journey toward becoming more competent in pharmacy communication, we hope that you will find the tools and strategies presented in this text to be useful. Communication is both a science and a form of art, as is patient-centered pharmacy care. As the profession of pharmacy continues to redefine its role and responsibilities in the new era of health care, it is crucial for our future generation of pharmacists to embrace the principles of patient-centered care and understand how effective communication plays an integral role.

REFERENCE

Howell, W. S. (1986). *The empathic communicator*. Prospect Heights, IL: Waveland Press.

GLOSSARY

Action stage of change is the stage in which changes are implemented.

Adherence is defined as the extent to which patients follow the instructions they are given for prescribed treatments.

Behavioral dimension of conflicts refers to our behaviors and actions during the conflict, and with these actions we express our emotions and manifest our cognitive processes related to the conflict.

Clinical empathy requires the provider's cognitive effort and ability to understand the patient's perspectives and experiences and to communicate that understanding and caring to the patient, without being misplaced in the patient's pain and emotions.

Coercive power comes with one's ability to punish or control.

Cognitive dimension of conflicts refers to the fact that conflicts essentially reflect our beliefs about values, needs, and goals, which are incompatible with those of the other party and cause the conflict.

Cognitive empathy occurs when one makes a conscious effort to recognize and understand the other person's emotional state, often referred to as *perspective taking*.

Collaborative relationship is a relationship with high provider control and high patient control, which closely resembles the concept of patient empowerment and is believed to be ideal for ensuring a truly collaborative relationship between the provider and the patient.

Communication competence is the ability to choose a communication behavior that is appropriate, effective, and ethical for a given situation.

Conflict is often defined as occurring between individuals with incompatible goals or needs.

Consumerist relationship is a relationship with high patient control and low provider control, in which the provider adopts a fairly passive role, acceding to the requests of an actively engaged patient.

Contemplation stage of change is the stage in which patients are ready to think about change and may recognize their behavior as problematic.

Cultural blindness is the stage in which all people are viewed the same without taking into consideration their cultural differences.

Cultural competence is the stage in which efforts exist for meeting the needs of diverse patients and customers, valuing diversity, and taking concrete steps to ensure efficacy in serving minority populations.

Cultural destructiveness is characterized by a complete lack of understanding of diverse cultures and an unwillingness to understand other cultures.

Cultural incapacity is characterized by a lack of capacity to respond effectively to culturally and linguistically diverse groups.

Cultural pre-competence is a very preliminary stage where strengths and areas of growth of cultural competence are known; however, progress has not yet been made to move forward.

Cultural proficiency is the active pursuit of resource development without hesitation.

Culture is a person's body of learned beliefs, traditions, and guides for behaving that are shared among members of a particular group. It involves all aspects of life, including values, beliefs, customs, communication styles, behaviors, practices, worldviews, clothing, art, and food preferences.

Defensive listening or aggressive listening is interpreting an innocent comment as a personal attack or a criticism and becoming defensive in the conversation.

Disability as contextually grounded refers to the definition of disability as a product of an interaction between a person's characteristics, such as physical abilities or social characteristics, and the environment's characteristics (built or natural).

Emotional dimension of conflicts refers to the emotional reaction to the cognitive dimension of the conflict; the emotions might be anger, fear, bitterness, frustration, hopelessness, or helplessness.

Emotional empathy, often referred to as *vicarious sharing of emotions*, occurs when we respond in a certain way, often subconsciously or unconsciously, to emotions displayed by others.

Empathy is the ability to understand the patient's experiences, pain, suffering, and perspective, and the ability to communicate this understanding and an intention to help.

Environmental barriers, also known as *external noise*, refer to anything in the physical or social background that makes effective communication difficult.

Expertise power refers to one's ability to influence others based on specific skills or knowledge.

Health literacy refers to the degree to which individuals have the capacity to obtain, process, and understand basic health information and services needed to make appropriate health decisions.

Information power is the possession of or access to information that others perceive as valuable.

Instrumental Goals are specific things you would like to accomplish with your communication, such as giving information to a patient.

Interprofessional collaboration is collaboration among members from different professions.

Interprofessional communication occurs when members of the healthcare team communicate in a collaborative manner for information exchange, collaborative decision making, and, ultimately, for attaining optimum patient outcomes.

Knowledge category of communication competence determines whether cognitively we can understand the communication dynamics and strategize which behavior is best suited for a given situation.

A **legally disabled individual** is someone who has a physical or mental impairment that substantially limits a major life activity, has a record of such an impairment, or is regarded as having such an impairment.

Legitimate power refers to authority associated with a position or one's title.

Limited English proficiency (LEP) individuals refer to people who do not speak English as their primary language and have a limited ability to read, speak, write, or understand English.

Maintenance stage of change ensures that the change in behavior becomes constant, with a focus on preventing relapse into old behavior.

The **medical model** of disability views persons with disabilities as individuals with physiological problems who need assistance or a curative solution to the problem.

Medication nonadherence includes delaying prescription refills, failing to fill prescriptions, cutting dosages, and reducing or changing the frequency of administration.

Motivation category of communication competence, which is shaped by our desires, interests, and values, ultimately determines whether we have the willpower to enhance our knowledge and improve our skills.

Motivational interviewing (MI) is a collaborative, person-centered communication style intended to elicit behavior change by helping patients explore and resolve ambivalence.

Noise is anything that interferes with the encoding and decoding of a message.

Paternalistic relationship is a relationship with high provider control and low patient control, in which the provider is dominant and decides what he or she believes to be in the patient's best interest while the patient assumes a more passive role.

Patient empowerment is defined as helping patients discover and develop the inherent capacity to be responsible for one's own life.

Perception-checking is a communication technique, where the pharmacist share his/her observation and perception of what is happening, describe what s/he considers to be the probable interpretations, and ask the patient for clarification to avoid misunderstanding.

Precontemplation stage of change is the stage in which the patient is not ready to think about change or is unaware that there is a problem.

Preparation stage of change is the stage of preparing for change.

Pseudo-listening is pretending to listen when we know we should be listening but feel we are unable to or simply cannot concentrate on the conversation.

Psychological barriers, also known as *internal noise*, include personal biases, perceptions, or other cognitive processes that interfere with our ability to effectively listen and contribute to a conversation.

Relational Goals refer to what we try to accomplish relationally with our communication, such as when we strategically communicate in a certain way to establish, maintain, improve, change, or at times terminate relationships.

Reward power comes with one's ability to give positive benefits.

Selective listening is listening to only parts of a conversation, usually the parts that interest us most.

Skill category of communication competence determines whether we have the ability and tools to enact the behavior in the given context.

The **social model** of disability views the disability not as a problem of the individual but focuses instead on the disadvantages he or she experiences in society as a result of these disabilities.

Unengaged relationship is a relationship with low provider control and low patient control and is not conducive to informed decision making by the patient.

Index

NOTE: Page numbers followed by *f,* or *t* indicate materials in figures, or tables respectively.

LEARN model, 68–69, 69*f*
    and patient communication, 65–69
    in pharmacy, 66–67
cultural destructiveness, 67, 67*f*
cultural incapacity, 67, 67*f*
cultural pre-competence, 67*f*, 68
cultural proficiency, 67*f*, 68
culture, 66

D
defensive listening, 147
dementia, 117
diabetes, adherence, 52
disability
    as contextually grounded, 129
    defined, 128
    perspectives on, 128–129
domains of pharmacy practice, 194

E
electronic health records (EHR), 196
electronic medical records, 10
elicit-provide-elicit model, 42
emotional dimension, 156
emotional empathy, 26
emotions, 158
empathetic listening, 27
empathy, 6, 26
    barriers to, 28
    and burnout, 28
    communicate, 27
engagement process of motivational interviewing, 40
environmental barriers, 28
communication, 145, 146
ethics and pharmacists, 8–10
evoke process of motivational interviewing, 41
expertise power, 183
external noise. *See* environmental barriers

F
federally assisted programs for LEP individuals, 81
focus process of motivational interviewing, 41
functional goals in interprofessional teams, 182

G
good communication, definition of, 7

H

I

K

L

language barriers, 80
language services
   for LEP patients, laws and regulations on, 81
   needs in United States, 80
Language Services Resource Guide for Pharmacists, The (NHeLP), 83
laws and regulations on language services for LEP patients, 81
LEARN model, 68–69, 69*f*
legally disabled individual, 128
legitimate power, 183
limited English proficiency (LEP)
   individuals, 80
   patients, 14
     laws and regulations on language services for, 81
     preparing pharmacy for, 83
     tools for communicating with, 81, 82*t*
low health literacy, patient communication, 91–95

M

maintenance stage of change, 39
medical model of disability, 128
medication adherence and patient communication, 51–55
medication counseling, effects on, 104, 105*t*
medication errors, 195
medication nonadherence, 52
   in older adults, 116
MI. *See* motivational interviewing
motivation, 8
   category, 7
motivational interviewing (MI)
   approach, biomedical approach vs., 38, 38*t*
   core communication skills of, 41–42
   four overlapping processes of, 40–41
   spirit of, 38–39
   stages of change, 39–40

N

National Assessment of Adult Literacy (2003), 116
National Council on Patient Information and Education, 104
National Health Law Program (NHeLP), 83
National Standards for Culturally and Linguistically Appropriate Services in Health and
     Health Care (National CLAS Standards), 66, 67, 81
Network for Excellence in Health Innovation report, 52
noise, 144
nonverbal cues, 196
   of empathy, 27

O

Office of Minority Health, National CLAS Standards, 66, 67
older patients, communication with, 115–118, 117*t*–118*t*

P

paternalistic relationship, 13
patient ambivalence, 38
patient care domain, 194
patient-centered approach, 14
patient communication, 166–167
  cultural competency and, 65–69
  medication adherence and, 51–55
  sensitive health topics, 168–169
  strategies for sensitive topics, 169–170
patient empowerment, 12–13
  approach, 14
Patient Protection and Affordable Care Act, health literacy defined, 91
patient-related factors, adherence, 53, 53*f*
patient-specific factor, 28
patient–healthcare provider relationship, 26
patient–provider relationship, 13
  modes of, 13, 13*t*
patients
  communication between pharmacists and, 156
  culture, 66
  with disabilities
    communication with, 127–131
    myths and facts, 129
  health literacy
    defined, 91
    facts about, 92
    influences health, 93–94
    myths about, 93
    tools for pharmacists, 94–95
    in United States, 92
perception-checking technique, 146
person-centered communication style, 38
personal/cultural barriers, patients with disabilities, 131
perspective taking, 26
pharmacist-specific factor, 28
pharmacist–patient communication, 196
  goals and ideals for, 6–7
pharmacist–patient relationship, 12, 14
  collaborative approach, 13–14
  patient empowerment, 12–13
pharmacists
  communication, 182–183

T

U

V

W